position**sex**

position**sex**

50 wild sex positions you probably haven't tried

lola rawlins

QUIVER

© 2007, 2011 Quiver

First published in the USA in 2007 by
Quiver, a member of
Quayside Publishing Group
100 Cummings Center
Suite 406-L
Beverly, MA 01915-6101
www.quiverbooks.com

The Publisher maintains the records relating to images in this book required by 18 USC 2257. Records are located at Rockport Publishers, Inc., 100 Cummings Center, Suite 406-L, Beverly, MA 01915-6101.

15 14 13 12 11   1 2 3 4 5

ISBN: 978-1-59233-507-7

Library of Congress Cataloging-in-Publication Data available

Book design by Michael Brock Design . www.mbrockdesign.com
Photography by Allan Penn

Printed and bound in Singapore

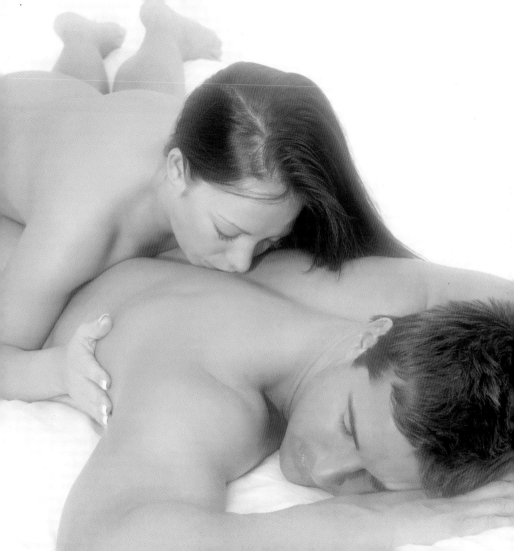

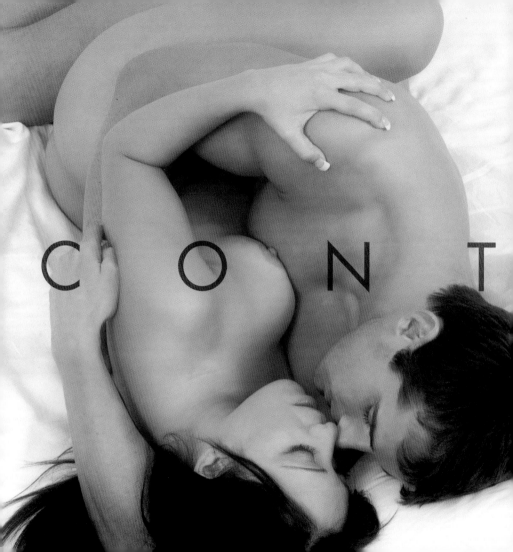

C O N T

E N T S

No. 1
LOCK & LOAD

A deep, undercover assignment.

HOW TO

Begin in the missionary position, but she should pull her legs in toward her chest, extending them so that her ankles hook on his shoulders. He then uses his hands to support both of their weight. Being extra flexible will allow both of you to enjoy the deep penetration and intense intimacy of this variation on your favorite standby. This position is great for a man with a shorter penis; however, if he is well endowed, thrusting can be painful for her, so be sure to communicate so you're both plunging to a pleasing depth.

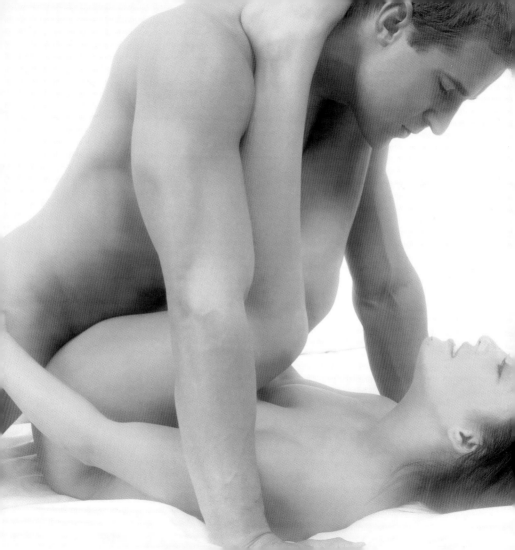

WHAT'S IN IT FOR HER

No matter the tenor of your sex session in this position, note that whenever you draw your knees to your chest, it shortens and tightens the vagina, so even shallow thrusts will make you tingle all over! Make sure you engage in ample foreplay before endeavoring to try this hot variation, because your man might not be able to hold out for long—the deep thrusting will drive him wild! Move into this position from something that was heating you up (an extra-long oral session, for example). If you're craving a connection with your man, this position can bring your lovemaking session to an extremely passionate place. Lock eyes and tell him how much you love him, or grab his hindquarters to pull him deeper into you.

WHAT'S IN IT FOR HIM

This position is all about deep penetration, and just when your woman thought you couldn't get any deeper, you lean forward and . . . WOW! Your balls will rest against her bottom, pleasantly stimulating an oft-ignored area. Placing pillows beneath her ass will also heighten your pleasure.

But aside from all the shoot-the-moon sensations of going deep with LOCK & LOAD, you will also love the feeling of control in this position. A woman's vulnerability can be a powerful turn-on for a man, so when she succumbs to your dominance, things will heat up even more!

No. 2
WIDE RELEASE

For his viewing pleasure.

HOW TO

The woman lies on her back, and the man kneels and enters her, holding a firm grip on her ankles and spreading her legs as wide as they can comfortably go. You'll want to experiment with the most pleasing width and pace of thrusting, as sensations can vary quite a bit.

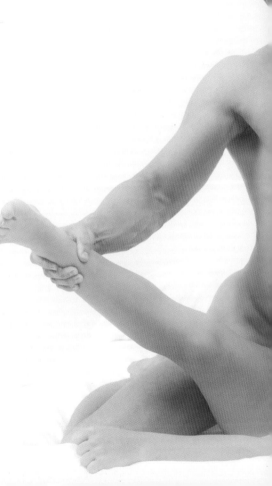

✳ WHAT'S IN IT FOR HER

Your hot bod is on full display! In this position, you're likely fulfilling one of his longtime fantasies, so revel in the fact that you are the star of the show. Penetration will be deep and the pressure of his pelvic bone on your clitoris adds delicious friction to the mix.

✳ WHAT'S IN IT FOR HIM

The turn-on for you in this position revolves around being able to see yourself insert your erect penis into her wet and willing vagina. The capability of men to become highly aroused from visual stimulation is well documented. Your lover will find immense gratification in knowing you're appreciating her naked and wide open body.

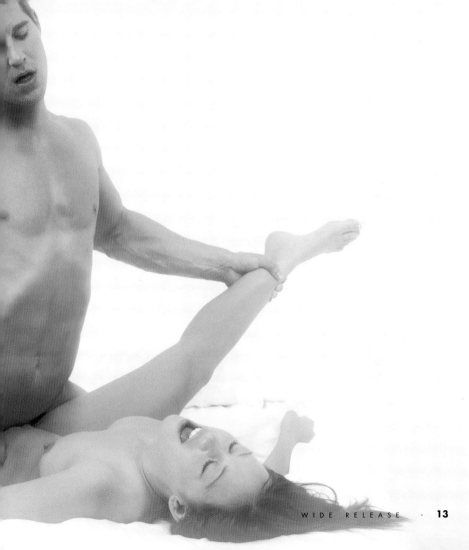

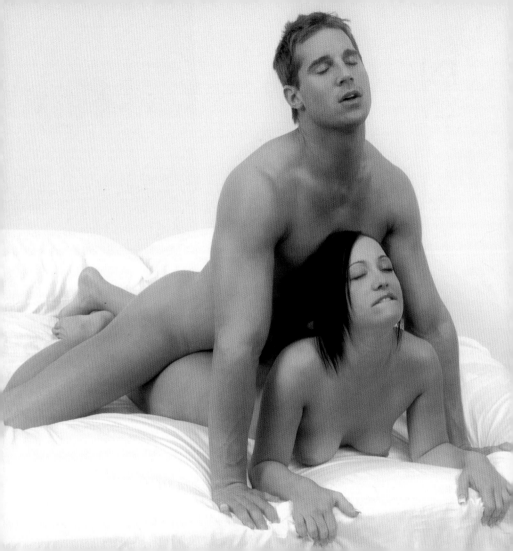

No. 3
THIGHS WIDE SHUT

A tight squeeze is all you need.

HOW TO

Lying face down on the bed, the woman rests on her elbows, with her legs parted just enough so that when her lover lies on top of her, he can slip inside. This might take some coordinated effort on both her and his part. Once he's in, she should squeeze her legs together. (For an even tighter grip, she should cross her ankles!) He supports himself with his arms and can either keep them extended for more exaggerated thrusting, or lower down to his elbows for some front-to-back skin contact and rhythmic, rocking action.

✂ WHAT'S IN IT FOR HER

THIGHS WIDE SHUT is perfect for deep thrusting, and you'll generate lots of friction with your legs closed tight. It's relatively mellow in terms of motion, but the sensations are amazing! (If he's prone to coming quickly, this is the perfect position to hold off climax until you're both ready to soar.)

By squeezing your legs together, you make the vagina feel longer and snugger, which is useful for accommodating a man with a large penis. The combo of lying face down and contracting the thighs stimulates the clitoris, which all but guarantees a stronger orgasm!

✖ WHAT'S IN IT FOR HIM

The pure, animalistic lust of rear-entry sex combined with the extra tightness of your lover's vagina makes this one for the record books.

"She gets off on being submissive, so I pin her hands down so she can't move and her breathing and moaning almost immediately becomes too much to handle!"

No. 4
BANANA SPLIT

A delicious treat between the sheets.

HOW TO

If you liked Position #3 (THIGHS WIDE SHUT), you're sure to find this tasty! The woman should lie face down on the bed, resting on her elbows. Once her lover slips inside, she slides her legs out very wide—so that they are almost perpendicular to her torso. He can remain higher up, supporting himself with extended arms, or he can drop down onto his elbows for extra contact. (If he lowers down, make sure the weight is comfortable for her. It's hard to get excited when you're being crushed!)

For an added jolt, she can loosen and tighten his pubococcygeus (PC) muscles to alternate sensations for him. (See Position #21, TIGHT DELIGHT, page 68.)

WHAT'S IN IT FOR HER

Extra-deep penetration and the feeling of friction on your pubic bone can send a spine-tingling jolt throughout your body, as your G-spot and your clitoris receive attention. Suggest a sexy mutual massage, complete with oil, before maneuvering into this position. This will provide a sweet, slippery sensation that only adds to the feeling of decadence.

WHAT'S IN IT FOR HIM

You get to go deep, deep, deep. And in the process, you get an amazing view of her backside. But if you can free a hand up during thrusting, and she feels comfortable with you exploring her nether regions, you will get a thrill out of teasing and fondling her anus. If your lover likes when you worship her behind, this will become her favorite after-dinner snack!

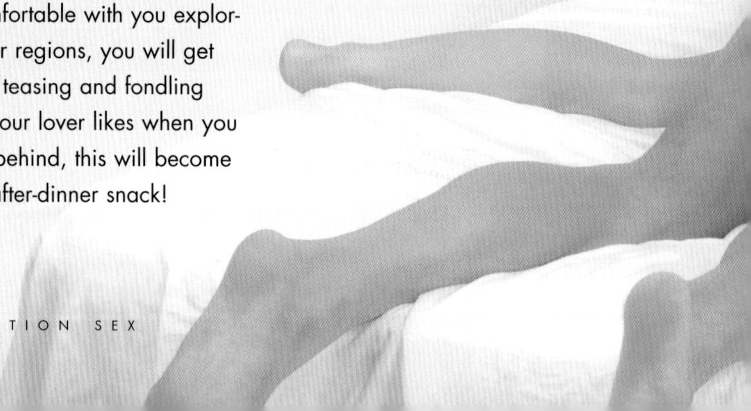

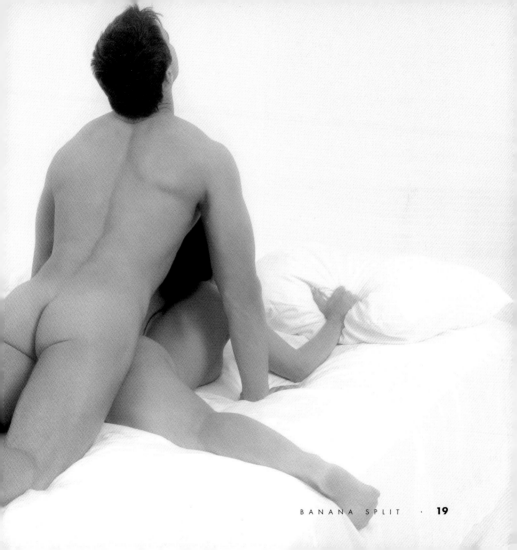

No. 5
RUMP ROMP

Boom, chicka boom!

HOW TO

She lies on her stomach or knees on all fours, while her lover kneels behind her. He can place his legs inside or outside of hers, and then he enters her from behind. This may take some coordination until he finds the right angle, and she'll need to experiment to find the right height for her hips for easiest entry into her vagina. Once he's in, the sky's the limit!

She may wish to close or tighten her legs to increase the friction and grip on his penis. He can thrust as slowly or as quickly as he likes, and either grab her hips or reach around and play with her breasts and clitoris. Deep thrusting is particularly easy, and the angle of penetration means the man can stimulate the upper inside wall of the vagina, where the G-spot is located—always a

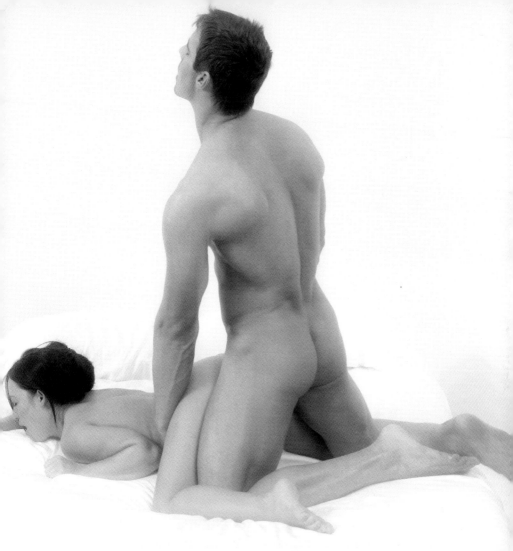

bonus! The intensity of the experience means he could come quickly, so this can be a good way to finish her sex session after she's reached her climax and he's ready to enjoy his.

✖ WHAT'S IN IT FOR HER

It allows deep penetration, which some women really enjoy! (Note that a RUMP ROMP can be overwhelming if your lover has a large penis.) In this position, his penis will likely stroke your G-spot, which bodes well for you achieving vaginal orgasm.

But your lover can also easily access your clitoris and play with it during sex for added ecstasy. If you want to play being "dirty" during sex, this position presents the perfect opportunity. You can really titillate your man by waving your ass around and acting raunchy!

✖ WHAT'S IN IT FOR HIM

Rear entry sex takes a man back to his lustful roots. It comes closest to sex as nature intended and gives you an outlet for your animal instincts. Seeing her bottom, with cheeks parted and your penis entering and withdrawing is almost too much stimulus for you! You will be uber-excited when taking her in from the rear, so don't be surprised if you come more quickly when having sex in this hot position.

No. 6

PILLOW

PLEASURES

On a pedestal of pillows.

HOW TO

This hot, lusty position is akin to RUMP ROMP—on steroids! Take the action off the bed and onto the floor as he prepares to worship her sexy body. The setup here is simple: Make sure one or two pillows are available. She stands on the ground, and bends over the bed leaning onto the pillows. The man faces the woman's back, comes right up next to her with legs slightly wider than hers, and enters her from behind.

✂ WHAT'S IN IT FOR HER

Unlike when he's on all fours, this position frees up his hands to fondle (or claw at!) your back and belly, massage your clitoris, gently tug your hair . . . . With a little imagination, the opportunities for heightened excitement are endless! You'll want to incorporate lots of foreplay, because in this position, he's so turned on, he may not be able to hold out for as long as he can in more tame entanglements. In addition to providing much-needed cushioning, the pillow can muffle your inevitable cries of ecstasy.

✖ WHAT'S IN IT FOR HIM

Any man will feel dominant and virile in this ultimate position of control. If you're especially fond of the view from behind, you're in the perfect stance to admire and play with her ass. With feet firmly planted on the floor, you can thrust with ease, control the tempo, and penetrate your lover oh-so-deeply! If you angle yourself up slightly, your balls will rub against her hind quarters each time you make contact for an added jolt of pleasure.

Choose Your Own Erotic Adventure

- Make it ultra intimate . . . by leaning over her and whispering in her ear; kissing and caressing her neck, touching and massaging her shoulders.
- Double the pleasure, double the fun . . . by teasing her! Slowly pull in and out of her AND enjoy the visual feast of seeing the penetration.
- Go a little harder . . . by thrusting with more gusto. The pillows will provide a soft bumper for her.
- Change it up . . . by varying the number of pillows that she has underneath her. Maybe you'll enjoy it with more, or maybe the hot spot is achieved with just one.

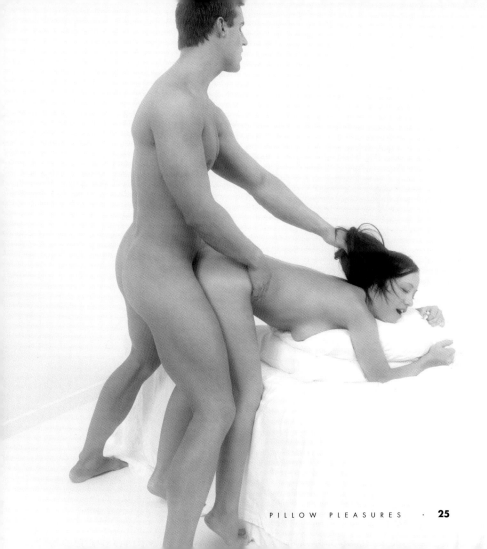

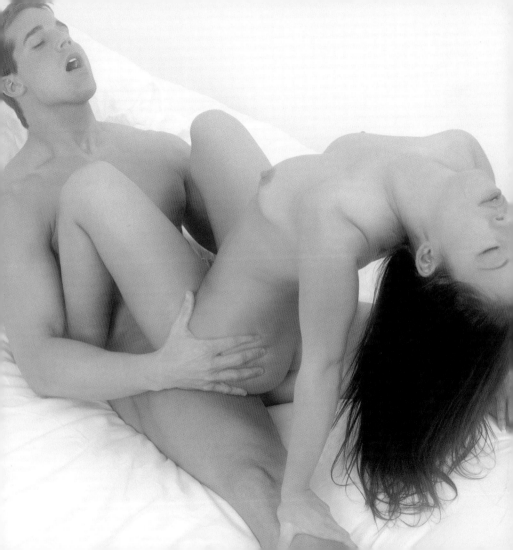

No. 7
SIT'N'SPIN

Anything but child's play!

HOW TO

Here's a position that's perfect for variations and experimentation. The man lies on his back, while the woman slowly squats onto his erect penis, positioning her feet near his hips and keeping her legs bent. (Be careful not to apply all of your weight at once!) She controls the action by moving up and down, rocking forward and back, or by gyrating her hips in a circular motion.

Up the erotic ante . . . by having her spin around! She slowly rotates to the side, and uses her hands and feet to keep herself stable. She then spins another 45 degrees so that her back is facing her man. She can either finish off in this position, or continue to rotate around so that their erotic encounter comes full circle!

✳ WHAT'S IN IT FOR HER

In this position, you call all the shots and you decide what tempo to set. If you're adventurous and enjoy taking the lead, you will love this lusty position. Penetration is deep, but you can also arrange for feel-good friction as you rotate around. This 360-degree delight also stimulates all the different areas of your vagina, so make sure to take the turn slow enough so you can make note of which angle really pushes your buttons!

If the idea of spinning makes you dizzy, swiveling your hips also ensures the head of your man's penis grazes every part of your inner walls.

✳ WHAT'S IN IT FOR HIM

You can sit back and enjoy the show, or can participate by using your hands to explore and caress, fondle and pinch, stroke, and stoke her flame!

"I like to masturbate after having sex with my husband, I'm still wet and his semen is smeared all around my sweet spot, which gets me even more hot!"

No. 8
SLICE OF HEAVEN

Forget about earthly pleasures …

HOW TO

In this position you get the tight fit of woman-on-top sex with the extra sizzle of doing it from behind! Start out with the man lying on the bed with outstretched legs. When he's ready, with her back to him, she squats over him and slides onto his hard penis. With knees splayed around his torso, she places her hands on his legs and takes her man for the ride of his life!

WHAT'S IN IT FOR HER

You're in control! This is one of the best ways for you to reach orgasm, because you determine the rhythm, speed, and depth of thrusting during the session. The angle of penetration is such that his penis will penetrate the front of your vaginal wall, which means you're in for some yummy G-spot stimulation. Drive your lover wild by grinding your ass into him. Then surprise him by taking matters in your own hands—literally. With SLICE OF HEAVEN, you are in the perfect position to access to your own juicy bits as well as his prized privates!

WHAT'S IN IT FOR HIM

Aside from the amazing view of her hot behind, your hands are free to roam, caress, fondle, and feel your lover up in any way that you please! It's like a dream for any man, especially because for the most part, he can just lie back and enjoy the ride. (Note that this might not be the most comfortable position for men whose erection normally stands upright against their stomach.)

G-Spot Giddyup!

Women have all heard about it, but have you been able to find this sometimes-elusive sweet spot? As it turns out, rear-entry and woman-on-top positions are best for its stimulation. To find your G-spot, spend some time exploring your body, and ask your man to lend a hand!

Insert a finger or two into your vagina, about two inches up, and then slightly crook them, making a "come hither" gesture. You'll be touching the front of your vagina. When you feel a small, button-sized spongy area, you've found it! Experiment with different pressures. As you stimulate it, the G-spot will often become more prominent as blood flows to the area.

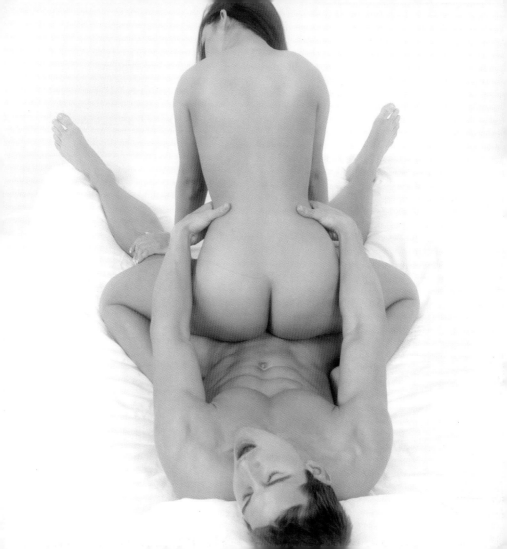

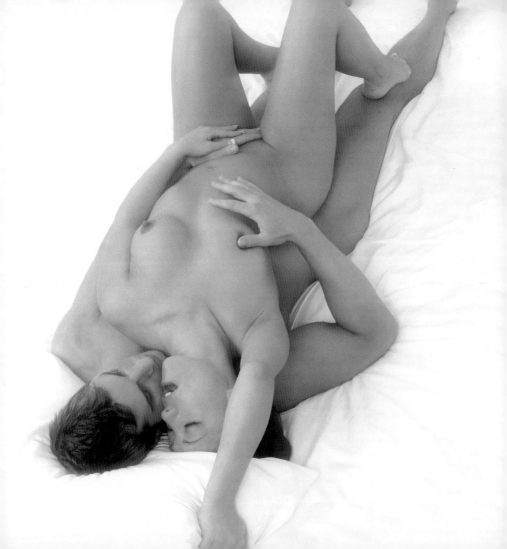

No. 9

BODY SURFING

Imagine you're at the beach.

HOW TO

The man lies on the bed with outstretched legs, while the woman faces his feet, and slowly lowers herself onto his erection. With his guidance, she slowly lies back, until she is resting on her lover's chest with her cheek near his. He should get the awesome sensation of her vagina lengthening as she lowers down on him. Slow and steadily, she pulls her feet up onto his legs and you ever-so-gently rock together to orgasm. This position is all about the deep feelings of small movements; he won't be able to move his pelvis, or she'll come apart.

✖ WHAT'S IN IT FOR HER

You've got to be pretty flexible to pull this position off, and the configuration requires some effort, but it's worth it! Whenever he penetrates you when your back is to him, his penis wakes up different regions of your vagina. This position can also be wildly passionate, as he's in perfect proximity to whisper in your ear, and kiss and nuzzle your neck. There's plenty of skin contact, which sends chemicals in the pleasure center of your brain soaring to create a feel-good glow you're not soon to forget!

✖ WHAT'S IN IT FOR HIM

You'll likely need both hands to keep her in position, but if you are both very balanced, you're free to focus your hands on her breasts and on exploring her clitoris. (You may even encourage her to masturbate so you know exactly where you should put your fingers.)

Since you're bearing all of her weight, you'll feel incredibly masculine (although this works better if you're taller or heavier than her)! Since her back is to you, this position could lend itself to playing out your fantasy scenarios. When she orgasms, you'll feel the amazing throb of her anus because your member is close to the wall of her vagina, proving to be an unforgettable erotic experience!

No. 10
OCTOPUSSY

Tangled up in you.

HOW TO

Here's a position perfectly suited for a long, slow, burning lovemaking session! The woman faces her man and gets in close. When heavy petting brings them both to the point of wanting to have intercourse, she should move in and open her legs just enough for him to enter by slinging a leg over hers. Another option for getting into this position: They start in missionary, and then they roll onto their sides, maintaining penetration as they rotate around. Enjoy the close and intimate feelings of making love while connecting with your eyes.

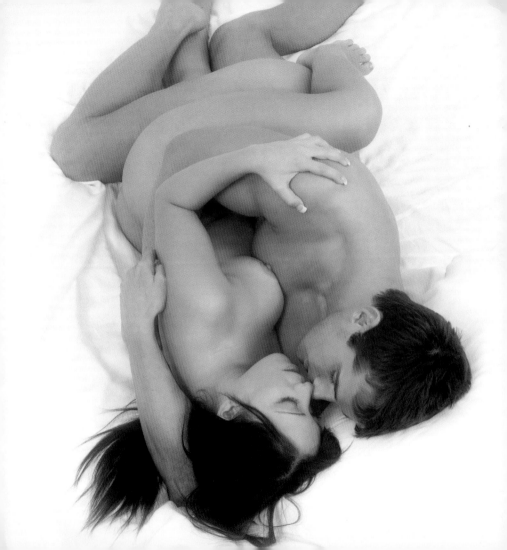

WHAT'S IN IT FOR HER

Here's a great way to delay orgasm: Tease your man by pulling your hips back almost to the point where his penis will come out and then plunge forward with a controlled thrust! The options for pleasure are only limited by your imagination: grinding, pelvic rotations and circular motions, tiny pulses, teasing, hands covering all the terrain . . . nothing's off-limits!

Side-by-side positions such as this are also ideal when you're sleepy, or if you're coming off a marathon of acrobatic sex and are craving just one more canoodle as a nightcap. Cuddly, but gentle sex provides a change of pace from thrusting and rhythmic routine. Don't separate too much, otherwise, you'll come apart from one another.

WHAT'S IN IT FOR HIM

If you're lucky, she'll send you over the edge by using her hands to wander to your perineum, the ultra-sensitive erogenous zone between your penis and anus. In this position, you can thrust gently and last for a long time before you come. Although hip movement is somewhat restricted, you can still get in deep, and if she wraps around you tightly, there is no danger of slipping out. If you're into breasts, you can nuzzle into her bosom, nibble her nipples, and derive a special kind of nourishment from her luscious orbs.

No. 11
V-O MAX

Lift your heart rate.

HOW TO

Time to show off your high kick! In this position, the man and the woman are on their sides facing one another. She lifts her top leg high into the air, and guides his erect penis into her wet vagina. He slides inside and wraps his top knee around her leg. Both of your hands are free to fondle and tease each other's sensitive bits. See how long you can hold the position before your leg tires!

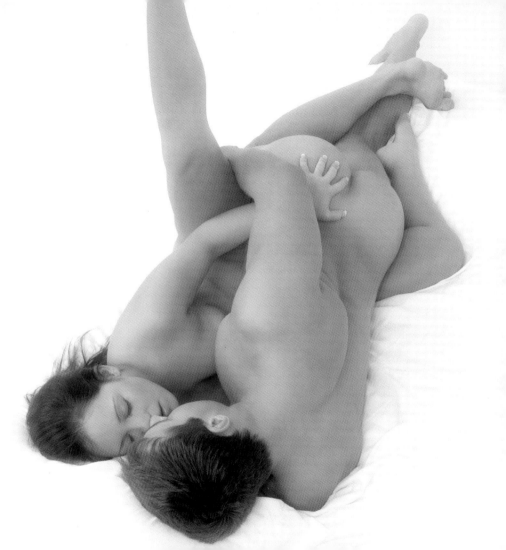

✖ WHAT'S IN IT FOR HER

Side-by-side positions are ideal for slow romantic lovemaking. This is a wonderfully intimate and connected position in which the partners can lie back and gaze into each other's eyes, or embrace closely and kiss, or just lie still while they enjoy the sensations of closeness. In this face-to-face position, the man can kiss and nibble his partner's breasts and she can see him do it, which can be a powerful erotic stimulus for her.

✖ WHAT'S IN IT FOR HIM

You can thrust gently and last for a long time before you come—movement of your hips is slightly restricted, but you can achieve good penetration. There is no danger of slipping out while you thrust because your partner can wrap her leg around you and hold you inside her while the lovemaking continues.

Lace Up Your Sneakers—For Sex!

You don't have to be a professional athlete to get the most out of sex, but there are proven stats that show the correlation between being fit and getting off! Aerobic activity revs up hormones, decreases stress levels, burns away fat, and rejuvenates the body, filling us with energy. A University of California study of middle-aged, sedentary men found that after just one hour of exercise three times a week, the men demonstrated improved sexual function, more frequent sex and orgasms, and greater satisfaction!

Since sex can be an act of endurance, improving cardiovascular fitness with aerobic activity such as walking, running, cycling, or swimming for at least thirty minutes, three times per week, will help both partners perform longer and more often.

No. 12
GIFT WRAP

Sealed in bliss.

HOW TO

When the man is sitting comfortably in a cross-legged or lotus position, the woman lowers herself onto his lap, wrapping her legs firmly around his waist and hooking her ankles in the back. She then slides onto his erect penis, and slowly leans backwards onto her outstretched arms. Don't speed through that last part, for there's a chance she could hurt her man, he could slip out, or both. When successfully executed, you'll both feel a tight, albeit shallow, penetration.

✖ WHAT'S IN IT FOR HER

Your man will rock you back and forth with a mesmerizing rhythm! You can vary the angle, reclining until you stop on a spine-tingling sensation. Your man can hold you in place with one arm and use the other to roam the front of your body—including your clitoris!

✖ WHAT'S IN IT FOR HIM

She controls the angle of penetration while you control the thrusting. Watch the temperature skyrocket as you pull her into you with great force, just as you're about to come. This feeds your animal instincts and heightens the intensity of orgasm for both of you!

Choose Your Own Erotic Adventure

The Lotus position is a classic yoga pose, and this is the underlying set up for GIFT WRAP. It's perfect for deep and intimate connection with your lover, as you gaze into each other's eyes and connect on a spiritual level. The focus here is not on thrusting—or even coming to orgasm! Your goal is to honor your partner by exchanging powerful and positive sexual energy.

Yoga and Sex

According to the Kama Sutra, "Pleasures are as necessary for the well-being of the body as food." And according to the tenets of yoga, sexual secretions contain the seeds of life and nutrients. Once there's depletion in life force, your vitality and ability to resist disease diminishes. Therefore, having a balanced and joyful sexual life is essential to your well-being! A complete branch of yoga, called Kundalini yoga, deals with harnessing sexual power. Through different yoga poses, you and your man can limber up, but more importantly, learn to take your lovemaking to a spiritual high ground.

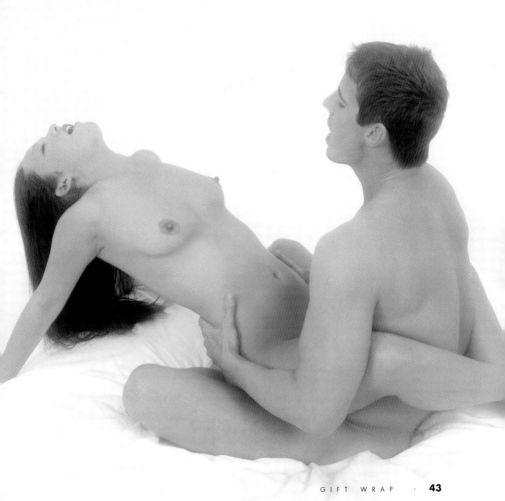

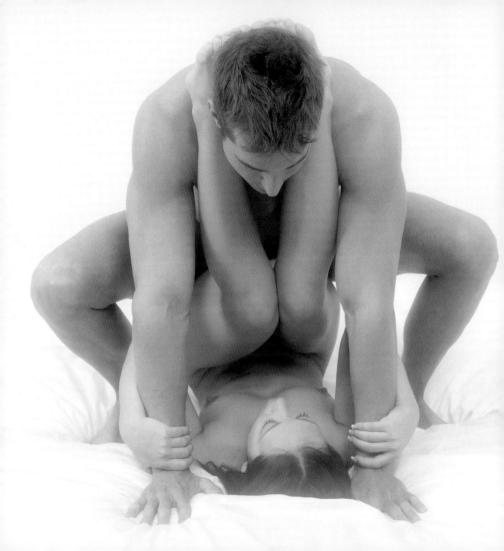

No. 13
CROUCHING TIGER

Sneak Attack!

HOW TO

After an enthusiastic round of foreplay, she lies on her back and while keeping her legs relatively tight, pulls them up towards her chest and into her body. Imagine a jungle scene as the man suddenly—and gingerly!—crouches over her, places his hands on the bed near her head, and slides into her. She hooks her ankles around his neck, and grabs his arms for added leverage and support. For a wild and randy ride, she can lift her ass to meet him for even deeper penetration. (For easier entry, she may also want to put a pillow under her bottom.) You can rock, but keep in mind that movement is mostly deliberate and controlled in this intense lovelock.

✂ WHAT'S IN IT FOR HER

If you're looking to connect in a carnal way, look no further. The unique configuration of this position lends excitement and novelty to your standard sex repertoire, but it still allows for intimacy. Because vigorous thrusting is abandoned in favor of slow, powerful contact, you and your man can lock eyes and talk to seal your bond. The angle of penetration means your man's bod will press against your vulva region, which can add to your excitement!

✠ WHAT'S IN IT FOR HIM

Because the woman is in a vulnerable position, you have the ultimate control in this dominant position. If she feels comfortable doing so, you can act out your domination fantasy! As part of this scenario, you may want to tease her by partially withdrawing for a few shallow thrusts, followed by a deep and forceful stroke. She might even follow your lead, and you both can witness an exciting new chapter in your sexual relationship.

No. 14
VIEW MASTER

He'll feast his eyes on this.

HOW TO

This starts out as the basic missionary position, but for the hottest results, the man should place a pillow beneath the woman's ass to raise her up; this allows for deeper penetration. Make sure her head is close to the edge of the bed. Once he's pumping, she can lift her arms and grasp the edge of the bed for added leverage. The motion of it all will turn him on, and she'll get a slight head rush, which makes her extra-tingly and amps up her excitement.

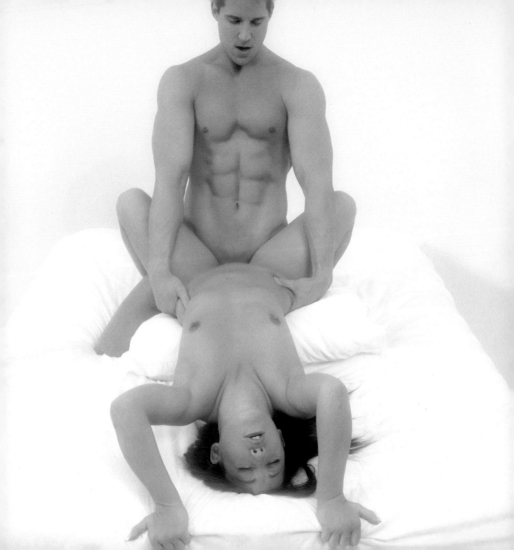

✂ WHAT'S IN IT FOR HER

Pushing against his pelvis adds friction to the equation, which presses all your pleasure buttons. When your man is lifting you and supporting your ass during thrusting, he can apply a little gentle pressure to draw your cheeks away from your anus and perineum, introducing a whole new erogenous zone and sending you over the edge!

✖ WHAT'S IN IT FOR HIM

This can be a position that affords delicious, deep penetration, but that's only true if you have a larger than average penis or a flexible erection. A man with a smaller penis, or one that points straight up when erect, is not likely to go too deeply into his partner with VIEW MASTER. If the latter is the case, you can relish the sexy sight of shallow bobbing in her wet and willing vagina. This visual will stay with you as a steamy mental image of your erotic adventures together!

Visual Turn-On

The brain is the body's most important sex organ. It gives and receives messages of desire through the eyes. The first spark of sexuality transmits unconsciously through the eyes. Later, the eyes become a conduit for desire—one look can set your lover aflame. Prolonged eye contact between two people is a potent sign of love and confidence. Pupil dilation is also an indication of attraction . . . . By letting your eyes roam across the body of your lover and linger on the genitals, you can give powerful clues about your intentions.

No. 15
UPSIDE-DOWN CAKE

Not for the faint of heart!

HOW TO

There are three ways to get into this amazing position: **HARD**—From Position #14 (VIEW MASTER), the man can move one leg so that it's bent and flat on the bed. Slowly, he pushes off that leg and rises up to a standing position, all the while keeping a firm grasp around her waist and trying not to lose penetration. Her hands are flat on the bed. When he's fully standing, she'll be in a backbend. **HARDER**—She starts out lying on the bed with knees bent, arms overhead, and hands placed by her ears. She arches her back and brings her hips high off the ground. The man kneels inside of her legs with

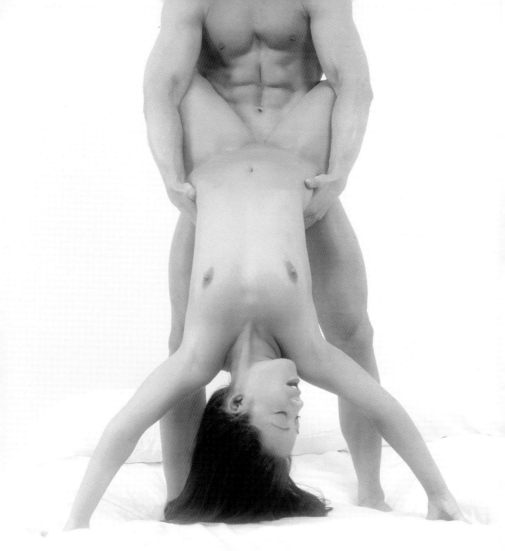

one foot flat on the bed, and grasps her around the waist to support the small of her back. When they're comfortable and ready, he raises up and lifts her off the ground. She wraps her legs tightly around his waist, while he gently enters her. **HARDEST**—If you're both extremely fit, you can get into this pose another way. From a standing position, the man lifts the woman into his arms and enters her as she straddles his torso, throwing her arms around his neck for support. From there, she lets go of his neck, clutches his forearms for support, and gradually lowers herself backwards until she can let go and place her hands on the ground in a handstand.

✵ WHAT'S IN IT FOR HER

This position represents an intimacy in your relationship. Face it: To pull this off, you and your man must trust each other and be in tune with each other's sexual energy. This can result in a mind-blowing orgasm for you as the blood flows to your head and your G-spot is stimulated.

✠ WHAT'S IN IT FOR HIM

Bragging rights! This acrobatic position allows you to show off your prowess. Note that this could be easier for you to accomplish after orgasm because the angle of penetration shortens the vagina and presses your member down.

No. 16
ALL THE RIGHT ANGLES

Factor in the feel-good friction.

HOW TO

She lies down on her back with her legs bent and apart. Her arms should be bent behind her shoulders. When the man is ready to enter her, he'll position himself between her knees and will raise her hips to meet his pelvis. She pulls herself up using her hands to support her raised back. To up the erotic ante, she should make sure her shoulders are on the edge of the bed and should throw her head backwards for a tingly head-rush!

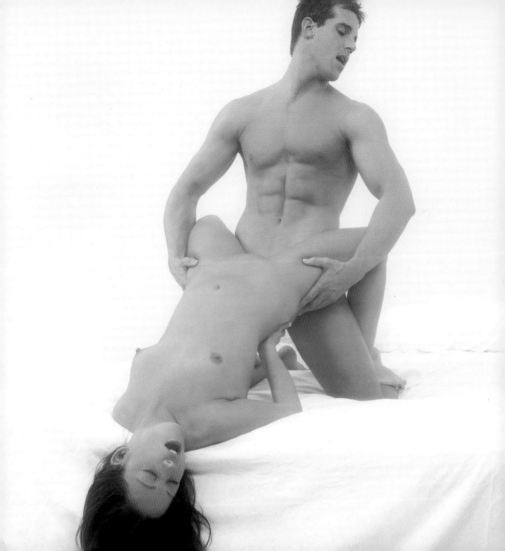

✂ WHAT'S IN IT FOR HER

As you move together in rhythm, you'll create friction that warms up your clitoris. Because of this, you'll likely experience more satisfaction than your man in this position. And although this can be a tiring position, it's worth the exertion because your man's penis is also angled up toward your G-spot. Talk about double the pleasure!

As if all that weren't enough, you can also stroke yourself while having sex in this position, and share control of the depth and force of penetration, by pushing further onto your man or pulling back.

✠ WHAT'S IN IT FOR HIM

Talk about a great view! And if your lover begins to touch herself? That will most likely put you over the edge! To take pressure off your balls, you should spread your legs (otherwise they could get squeezed).

Does Size Matter?

According to an informal study done in early 2006 by editors of *Cosmopolitan* and *Men's Health*, women are overwhelmingly more interested in her lover's thrusting and oral sex techniques than his penis girth or length. And when it comes to size, 64 percent of those polled said the ideal girth of their man's member was "as big as a D battery." The takeaway? It's not what you have, it's how you use it!

No. 17
BACKSEAT DRIVER

Revved for action!

HOW TO

He is sitting with his knees in tight and tucked beneath him. She is kneeling in front of him so that their bodies are tucked closely together. She rubs her bottom in the area of his genitals to heat him up and then slides on top of him when they're both primed for action! This is a great position if you only have time for a quickie, or if you are looking for a rear-entry position with greater potential for intimacy.

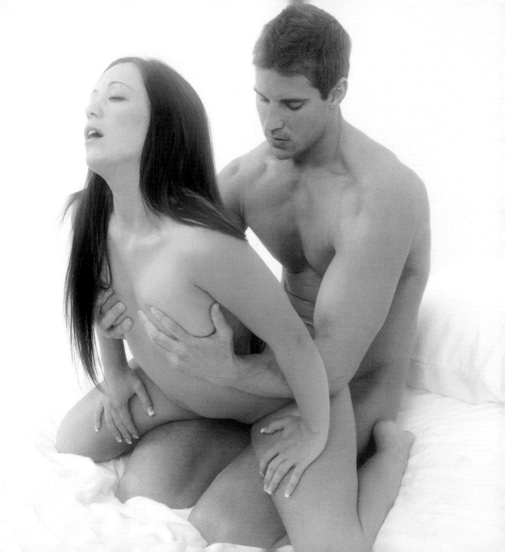

✣ WHAT'S IN IT FOR HER

He may be in the driver's seat, but . . . you have the keys to take this beauty out for a joy ride! This can be a more restful position, and you can control the tempo and tenor of the lovemaking session, either moving quickly or slowly, thrusting your hips up and down, in a circular pattern, or in a gentle rocking motion. This position offers good G-spot stimulation; for even deeper penetration, open your legs wide. Add some oomph as you're about to come—reach behind and grasp his back to pull you both extra tight!

✠ WHAT'S IN IT FOR HIM

Your hands are free to roam her body, and you may want to lavish extra attention on her breasts. If you sync up with her motions, the friction and rhythm can send you both soaring! Since you're both on your knees, you might be more comfortable with cushions beneath you (especially if you decide to take this move from the bedroom to the stairwell!).

Breast Behavior

Guys, a note of advice: Don't breast-feed, bite, chew, or act as if you're tuning a radio. Instead, treat breasts like they're soft serve ice cream cones. Use gentle kisses, caresses, long licks, and strokes all over both breasts and take your time! Remember, women are touchy about their breasts (similar to how men are sensitive about their penis girth), so if you're going to comment, focus on their beauty, not their size.

No. 18
LUSTY
LAYBACK

Ride him, cowgirl!

HOW TO

From Position #8 (SLICE OF HEAVEN, page 29), she can show her flexibility and maneuver into this position by leaning back and grabbing onto his ankles. He continues to grasp her waist to control the movements, which can get pretty intense!

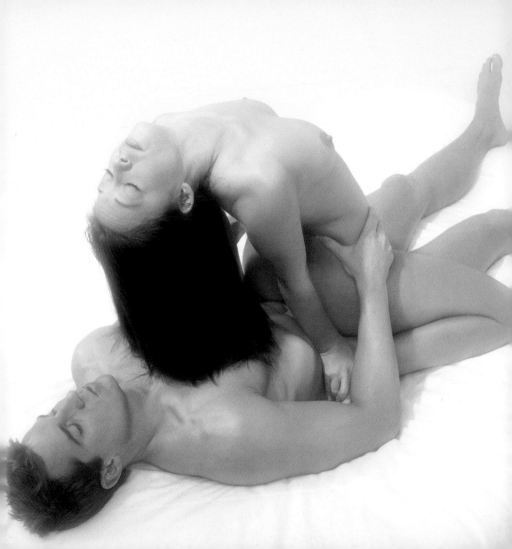

✂ WHAT'S IN IT FOR HER

Feeling dominant? Then this is the perfect position to impart your power! You control the depth, intensity, and angle of penetration, while he submits to your every wish. Slow, controlled movements work best, and circular motion will get him buzzing. Deep penetration will massage your G-spot, and if you're able to free up a hand, your clitoris may also benefit from some pointed pressure!

✳ WHAT'S IN IT FOR HIM

Enjoy the relaxing opportunity of reclining as you let her set the tempo! And since you can't see her face, you're free to let your fantasies take flight . . . Perhaps you'll address her as if she is a stranger. Go with it, and you'll be excited to discover that this kind of "dirty" talk can ratchet up the heat in your bedroom!

You can also caress the front of her body, play with her bottom, or reach around to finger her sweet spot. Note that since your penis is bent down in this position, you should take care that if it slips out during intercourse it isn't hurt.

"Talk Dirty to Me"

Erotic talk happens to be one of the most powerful forms of seduction. It can make your love life racy and more creative. It can help you form a deeper bond with your partner and opens the lines of communication in the bedroom. Your only limit is your imagination!

One couple recounts what happened when they became more verbal during sex: "We began making more erotic declarations, not the 'fuck me fuck me' of porn, but things like: 'I love the way you suck/lick me.' Or 'Roll over. I want to fuck you from behind.' Or 'Stick your tongue inside me.' Erotic talk became a real turn-on for both of us."

No. 19
SITTING PRETTY

A lusty lap dance.

HOW TO

He sits up on the bed, leaning against the headboard for support. She faces him, and lowers herself onto his erect penis, leaning back for support, resting her hands on the bed or grasping her man's lower legs. With his help, she raises her legs up one at a time and rests them on his shoulders. In this position, movement will most likely be limited. He cradles her lower back for support, and both lovers will find bliss by either rocking in sync together or he can take the reins and pump his love muscle until they're both in a frenzy.

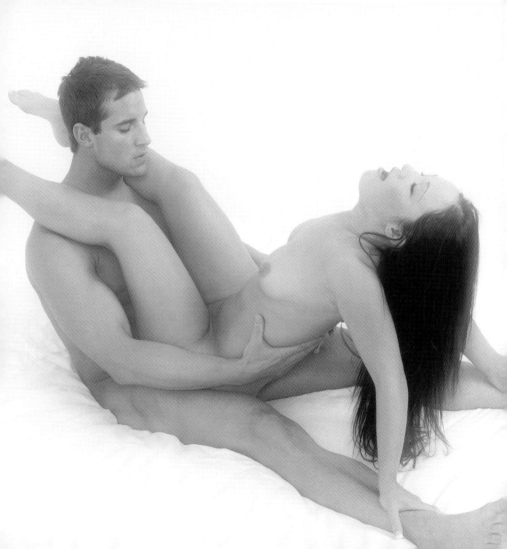

WHAT'S IN IT FOR HER

If intimacy is what you're after, this position provides plenty of opportunity for variation: Instead of leaning back, wrap your arms around your lover's strong arms and get close enough for passionate kissing and lots of touching. In this closer variation, lovemaking is slow and sensual, and could free up your lover's hand to roam to your sweet spot! Either way, because penetration is deep, you have a better chance of reaching vaginal and clitoral orgasm.

WHAT'S IN IT FOR HIM

You can relish in the highly erotic nature of this pose, especially if she consciously flaunts her body for you. You will quickly get off on the visual feast she's serving up! In addition to seeing her in an open state, you have a perfect view of her bobbing breasts and the motion of penetration, both of which are an unbelievable turn-on for any hot-blooded male! You may feel inspired to talk dirty to ratchet up the excitement and help fuel your wildest fantasies.

Make Size Matter

Ninety-five percent of men measure the average five to seven inches when erect, but if he falls outside this range, here's how you can maximize your passion potential.

- If you're underfunded, go for deep-penetrating woman-on-top positions (especially variations that have you facing your man, but leaning backwards).
- If you're overendowed (there IS such a thing, and it can hurt!), he needs to hold back and ease slowly. You need to let him know when you're ready for a harder and faster ride.

No. 20
HIGH HEELS

A rush of blood to the head ...

HOW TO

She lies back on the bed, and gets into position to do a shoulder stand, with just her upper back and shoulders touching the bed. Her lover kneels in close to her and enters her as he rests her legs up against his torso. A little coordination is necessary to achieve penetration, but once you've figured out the alignment, hold on tight, because you're in for a deep ride!

✖ WHAT'S IN IT FOR HER

You've got to be extra supple and flexible for your body to withstand this position for any length of time (in fact, HIGH HEELS is a great abdominal workout!), but there are blissful benefits for you. Anytime your legs are up, you will experience deeper penetration during sex, meaning that your man's member will hit all the juicy spots in the back portion of your vagina. That, combined with the amplified pleasure when blood rushes to your head during orgasm, will leave you feeling giddy!

✖ WHAT'S IN IT FOR HIM

You have to be blind to not enjoy this vista! (If she slips on a pair of sexy stockings and stilettos, she will really drive you over the edge!) As it requires a bit of deliberate movement to get into this position, it's not likely one she'll find herself in often, so you'll be especially turned on by the unique view of her elongated body. The deep penetration ensures that every inch of your penis is receiving stimulation.

Primed for Action

Many people find the sight of their partner masturbating highly erotic. It can also be very instructive to discover how your partner reaches orgasm alone, as this will be the best method for you to adopt when you are touching him or her. Masturbating with your partner will break down inhibitions and allow you to get even closer.

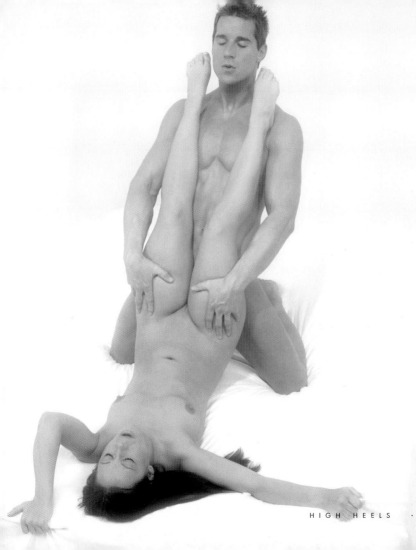

No. 21
TIGHT DELIGHT

Squeeze to please.

HOW TO

This is a twist on the missionary position, whereby once he has entered her, she pulls her legs together tight, essentially sandwiching his penis and adding delicious friction with each thrusting motion.

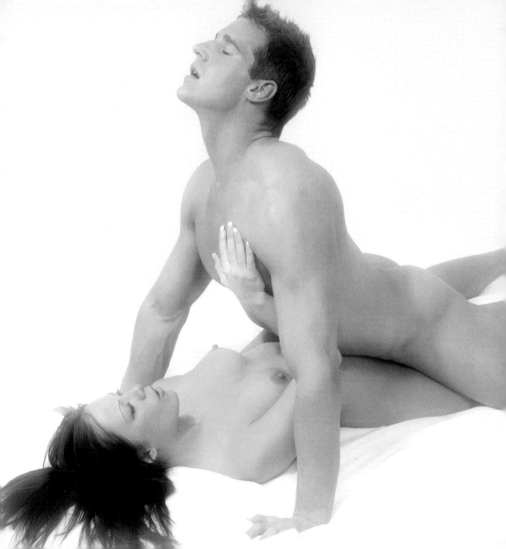

✂ WHAT'S IN IT FOR HER

You finally get to put your Kegel exercise training to good use! A tight squeeze and more genital contact means that each time he thrusts, the pressure of his pelvis and angle of entry will stimulate your clitoris and the sensitive nerve endings in the outer regions of the vagina. This is an excellent position to move to after you've already reached orgasm, because there's a good chance your man won't be able to hold out for long!

✳ WHAT'S IN IT FOR HIM

The tight, warm grip around your penis will have you throbbing in ecstasy in record time.

CAT's in the Bag

Here's a variation on the missionary position that's intimate and truly sensational! Coined by sex researcher Edward Eichel, Coital Alignment Technique, or CAT, involves the man positioning himself slightly higher so that the base of his penis makes contact with the woman's clitoris when he enters her. It's more about vibration than thrusting. When she wraps her legs around her man, places her feet on his calves, and stretches her legs slightly, she also helps her clitoris find its way to her lover's penis. The end result? She'll be stimulated internally and externally.

Coordinated movement is the key to this rhythmic, rocking technique. Penetration is shallow and the result is a series of very small collisions. If you practice the slow, sensual crescendo of these rhythmic movements, you'll soon realize this position is designed for a big finale!

No. 22
SPOON BENDER

Make mine with a twist.

HOW TO

Get into the traditional spooning position: The man lies on his side with knees bent, and she also lies on her side with knees bent and her back pressed against his front. She parts her legs slightly and aligns his penis with her vagina for easy entry from the rear. She twists her upper body around to complete the spoon bender.

✄ WHAT'S IN IT FOR HER

Full-body contact makes for highly intimate, gentle lovemaking. If you're a bit tired from a high-octane session earlier in the evening, this is a sweet way to wind down. Penetration is shallow, so he should be able to go for quite some time in this relaxed position. By twisting toward your man, you can look each other in the eye, and you give him easier access to your breasts and clitoris.

✳ WHAT'S IN IT FOR HIM

Before you enjoy the warm, wet feeling of being inside of her, you can tease her and arouse yourself by moving your penis in and around her buttocks. Squeezing your penis between her cheeks will simulate penetration and make you ache for more. Once inside, this position offers an opportunity for you to fondle her breasts, nuzzle her neck, whisper seductively in her ear . . . . All of these things make you even more endearing to her, and tightens the bond between you. When she twists around, you can bite and tease her nipples, and take in the view of her outstretched body.

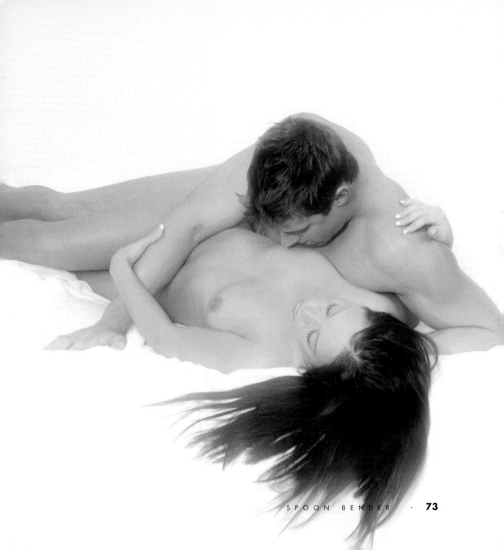

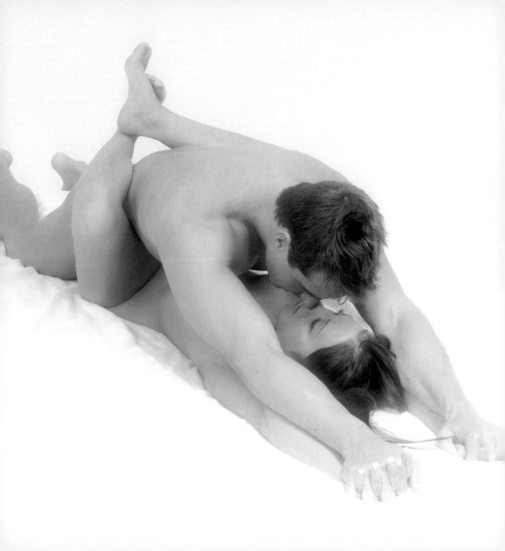

No. 23
POWER PLAY

Where do you think you're going?

HOW TO

Here's a highly erotic spin on the missionary position. He mounts her as he would in the old standby, but in doing so, he pulls her arms up over her head and either holds her wrists together or lightly pins her arms down on the bed. She pulls her legs up around his back to meet his thrusting and so deepens the experience.

✂ WHAT'S IN IT FOR HER

If you have always wondered about incorporating this type of play into your bedroom repertoire, look no more! Here's a perfect entrée into light bondage. You'll get off on his taking control of the situation. Of course, your man won't hurt you, but the feeling of being trapped could awaken latent fantasies for you. Use dirty talk to explore your desires! Keep in mind that with your legs raised around his back, you still retain some control. For added spice, pull his ass into your body by squeezing him tight.

✕ WHAT'S IN IT FOR HIM

The thrill of domination! Understanding that as a sexual partner, you trust each other enough to explore edgier ways to fulfillment.

Intro to Bondage

If you are looking for a very basic introduction to light bondage that's presented in a cute, nonthreatening way, look no further. Vanilla Bondage is a whimsical "submissive lover's kit" packaged like a pint of ice cream and topped with suggestions of how to make your "vanilla" fantasies more kinky. This carton of fun contains one cream-colored blindfold and two ribbon-like tethers. It is designed more for the novelty of trying out light bondage than getting down and dirty with heavy S/M.

No. 24
DOWNTOWN TRAIN

All aboard the Erotic Express!

HOW TO

The action extends from the bed to the floor in this randy romp! She positions herself so that the lower half of her body (from her waist down) is on the bed and her arms are on the floor supporting her upper body, which is angled down. Her ass is right on the edge of the bed, and her legs are spread open. He pulls into the station and slides in from behind. He supports his body weight by extending his arms and grasping the edge of the bed.

✂ WHAT'S IN IT FOR HER

As this position requires a bit of upper-body strength, you'll need to have your man experiment with tempo so that your lovemaking session is enjoyable and not unduly strenuous. If you're looking to move from tame on-the-bed entanglements to more acrobatic adventures, take the DOWNTOWN TRAIN to make the transfer! Adding a pillow under your waist will add extra feel-good friction and all but guarantee G-spot stimulation. You'll feel extra buzzy as blood flows to your brain, making your climax even more intense!

✠ WHAT'S IN IT FOR HIM

You direct the off-the-rail excitement! You'll love the feeling of control, as you pump until she can't take it any more. By just sliding to the edge of the bed, she adds a truly thrilling twist to sex. You'll get off on the novelty of the position as well as the view from the conductor's seat!

"We were walking home from the bar, and he just scooped me up in his arms, kissed me, and carried me the rest of the way home. It was only about ten yards, but the gesture was there. We had unbelievable sex the second we shut the door."

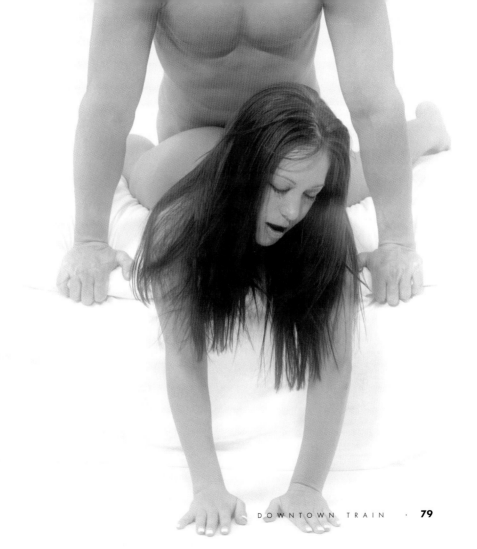

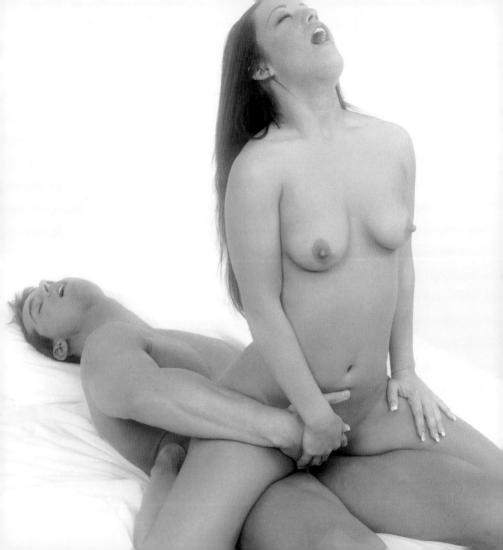

No. 25
CLIT CONTROL

Press that magic button.

HOW TO

He lies on the bed and with her back to him, she slides on top of his stiff shaft. She bends her knees and places her feet behind her. She leans back slightly so that her crown jewel is easily accessible and schools him in the fine art of pleasuring her!

✂ WHAT'S IN IT FOR HER

You can control the tempo and intensity of thrusting. The angle of the position means his member will hit your G-spot. Moreover, you—and your man—can focus on giving you a mind-blowing orgasm by spoiling your sweet spot (i.e., stimulating your clitoris)! If you time things right, you can come together! At that moment, grind your hips down into his pelvis for ultra-hot sensations!

✖ WHAT'S IN IT FOR HIM

As she leans back, your penis goes extra deep. Although this seems like a passive position for you, you can relish in the fact that by pressing the right buttons, you can drive her wild!

When I Think About You, I Touch Myself

Here's a quick lesson for him on navigating her pleasure nub, affectionately referred to as her clitoris.

ROLLING Place a thumb and forefinger around the nub and gently roll it in between his fingers. Start off gently and gradually apply pressure and speed the pace based on her feedback.

ROUNDING He can make her come quickly with this method! She takes his first two fingers and places them over top of her clitoris. Move them in a circular motion and vary the speed and pressure. Wet fingers work best!

TAPPING This two-handed technique is a little different and produces exceptional orgasms! He should use his left hand to pull the lips back out of the way so that her clitoris is exposed. With the index finger on his right hand, lightly tap the clitoris. Sensations build until she just can't take it any more, as he becomes an expert at getting her off.

No. 26
PRIMAL PUMPING

Pouncing pleasure.

HOW TO

Similar to Position #5, RUMP ROMP, but with added animalistic eroticism. She crouches down on her knees with her arms outstretched (she can grasp the edge of the bed for support). In a swift move, the man enters her from behind, while leaning his arms on the bed. He can pull his knees open wide for more leverage to thrust oh-so-deep!

✂ WHAT'S IN IT FOR HER

The carnal nature of the pose brings you back to basic urges and feels just right if you're both in the mood for an impersonal and rougher session in the sack. As with all rear-entry positions, he can push well into you, so make sure the pressure is pleasurable, not painful. With your legs pulled into such a compact position, the added friction you feel when his privates hit your wet mound with each thrust is truly delicious!

✠ WHAT'S IN IT FOR HIM

Lustfulness is the driving force behind this position. You are master of your domain, and you want to take her from behind—and take her authoritatively! The sense of power combined with the exaggerated sensations that result in a tight squeeze around your throbbing member will send you over the edge, and quick! The urgency around this position prevents it from being a drawn-out nookie session.

The Penis Parade

Every year on March 15, Japan throws a giant festival to celebrate the penis and fertility. A 900-pound wooden phallus is paraded around the streets of the town Komaki, and women carry massive dildos in their arms. Thousands of people come to pay homage to the penis and take part in the festivities.

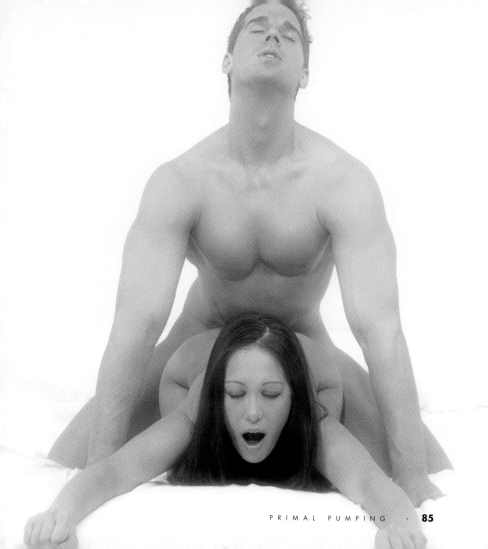

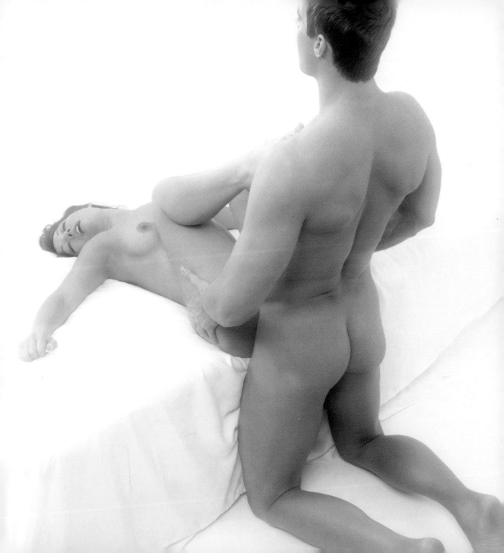

No. 27
LIKE A PRAYER

Time for a true confession …

HOW TO

When he kneels at the altar of her sexuality, he's a changed man! She lies back with her ass near the edge of the bed. He kneels on the floor close to the edge of the bed and pulls her bent legs up to his chest. (He can put pillows under his knees to make this position more comfortable or to adjust the height.) As he gently lifts her bottom, he slides his erect penis inside of her. The result is a religious experience!

WHAT'S IN IT FOR HER

When he plays with your ass, there's great potential for arousal. This compact pose can be made even more heavenly if you contract and release your PC muscles intermittently for an even tighter fit. While he sets the tempo, you can push against his chest and raise your bottom to meet his thrusting to add to the naughtiness. This is another good position to ease you into the next level of adventurous lovemaking.

WHAT'S IN IT FOR HIM

Visual stimulation is a powerful turn-on for men, and in this position, you can feast your eyes on your erect member plunging into her willing vagina. The excitement of that combined with the pleasure that comes when she pushes against your chest (which deepens the angle of penetration) will have you throbbing in no time. The memory of this session in the sack will promote dirty fantasies that will stay with you until your next confession.

No. 28
CORKSCREW

I'd like that on the side, please.

HOW TO

She lies on her side with her legs close together and bent at the waist (her body should almost form an L-shape). She lets her head fall back on the bed, and opens her legs slightly to allow her man to enter her from behind. Similar to Position #22, SPOON BENDER, on page 71, but with one special twist: Once he's inside, she squeezes her thighs tightly together for added friction. Crossing her legs at the ankles will help her keep them closed shut! The movement here is intense—slow, gentle, and coordinated.

✄ WHAT'S IN IT FOR HER

If you have difficulty coming without clitoral stimulation, this is a great position for you! When your legs are closed tight, you'll feel the tingly sensations that are inevitable when your magic button is rubbed. In fact, the leg-lock could cause your entire pelvic area to hum. The rear-entry penetration is not so much deep as it is tight, but sweetened by forward-facing intimacy and visual stimuli of seeing your man over you! As he's entering you at a unique angle, he'll stimulate a new region of your vagina. Notice the new sensations!

✵ WHAT'S IN IT FOR HIM

It's going to feel so otherworldly and you're going to want to thrust vigorously, but in doing so, you run the risk of slipping out. Instead, you're better off using very controlled movements to savor every moment inside of her in this tight pose. Her thigh lock extends her vagina—as well as the pleasure you feel with each well-positioned thrust!

For a better view of her body, and to alter the angle of penetration, you can pull yourself into a more upright position, using her bottom to support yourself. This slight variation means heightened enjoyment all around as you press her ass to deepen your thrusts.

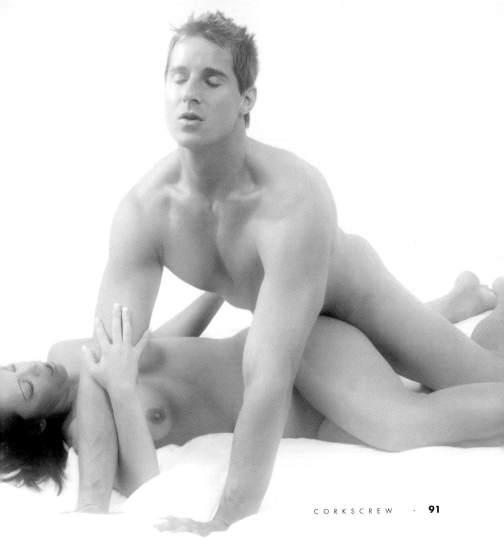

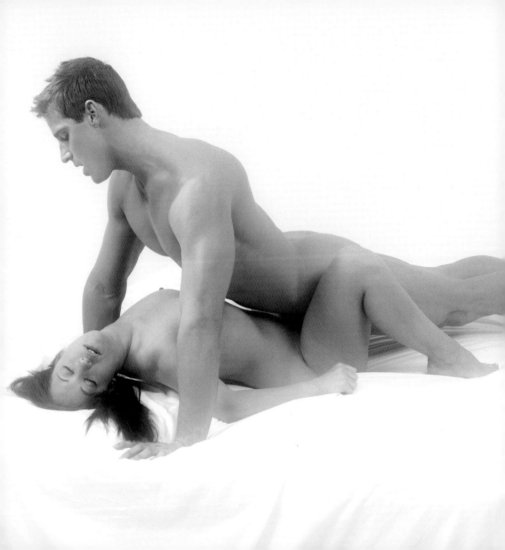

No. 29
TRISEX DIPS

A carnal core workout.

HOW TO

If he works hard to stay fit, this can be a sexy way for him to show off his rock-hard abs and arms while teasing her into submission! She lies on her back on the bed as he positions himself above her, as if he's going to do a push-up, balancing on the balls of his feet with legs taut and his arms fully extended near her head. As he slowly lowers himself, he uses his pelvic region only to guide his erect penis into her. Balanced and controlled contact is how this position plays out, as he purposely keeps his body away from hers.

✄ WHAT'S IN IT FOR HER

The kink factor here revolves around the game of genital-only contact. Agree ahead of time that you will not grab his ass, throw your legs around his torso to pull him in tighter, or reach out to squeeze and bite his toned pecs. Instead, up the erotic ante by giving him a verbal stream of commentary about what you'd like to do to him, describing each move that you're *not* actually doing in great detail. See how long each of you can hold out. If you have more willpower, you can make the rules for your next randy romp!

✄ WHAT'S IN IT FOR HIM

This position is deceivingly simple. When she's in such a vulnerable state, it's a challenge for you to keep away from her. It's going to take every fiber of your being to resist mauling her, especially if your lovemaking sessions are normally full of heavy petting and lots of touching. But this affords her the opportunity to concentrate on the sensations that build around her pelvic region when very small movements are made. You will tease her until she can't take it anymore, and that makes you feel virile and dominant.

No. 30
STANDING O

We're reaching for the stars ...

HOW TO

This ambitious position may be difficult for some couples to accomplish, but it's amazing what can happen when you experiment and practice at it! This obviously works better if you are a similar height. Stand close to one another with the man behind. He'll need to spread his legs to a width that puts his penis in line with the opening of her vagina. When you're both ready, he'll glide his erect member into her, relishing the view. He'll likely need to use his hands to do this. Once he's inside, he can raise her arms overhead and clasp hands with her. Coordinated movement is essential to finding bliss with this STANDING O.

WHAT'S IN IT FOR HER

The challenge here is in remaining penetrated. You'll find that the inability to move will add an extra spark to your arousal. But there are many variations if you find this too difficult to maintain or if you are a lot shorter than your man. You can reach for a door jamb to give you both added leverage. You can lean against a wall and his hands can grasp your waist to pull you into him while thrusting. A stairway may level the playing field, as you can go a step higher, which should put your genitals at the same height for easier penetration.

WHAT'S IN IT FOR HIM

Because of the lack of stability in this position, penetration will be shallow. Once you're inside of your lover, you may want to stay there, and experiment with small circular motions and lateral jerks, as opposed to typical in-and-out thrusting. This may make you vulnerable to premature ejaculation because of the unique angle (the head of his penis is rubbing her inner body in such a way that it will be hard for you to control your orgasm). This position is best used for quickies!

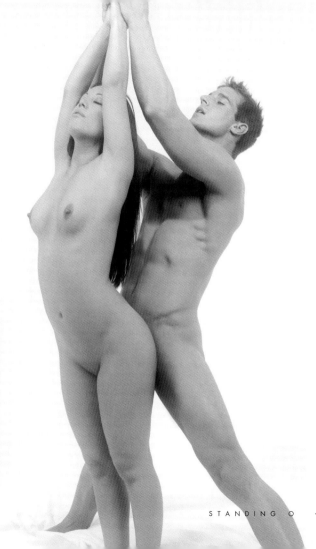

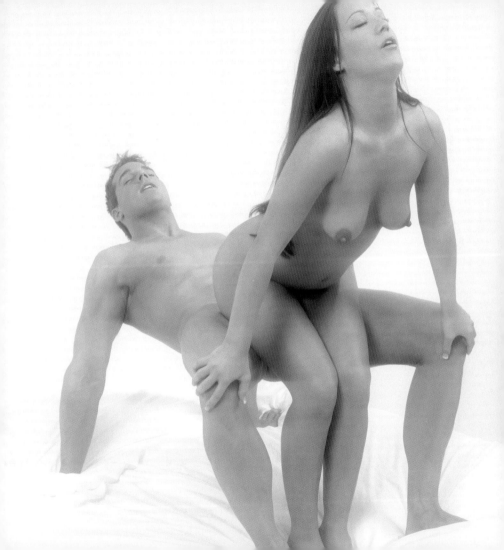

No. 31
LAP OF LUXURY

He's no Lay-Z-Boy!

HOW TO

Here's a unique way to get it on—one in which the man gets a workout at the same time. He moves into a bridge-like position, with legs and arms planted firmly on the bed with his body raised so that his torso is almost entirely flat, like a table. With her back to him, she slowly sits onto his erect penis, keeping her bent legs together tight and placing her hands on his thighs for stability. She's in for an exciting ride in this decadent position!

WHAT'S IN IT FOR HER

The novelty of this is something that will stay with you for quite some time. The angle allows for lots of G-spot stimulation, always a good thing! And the friction created from your legs being closed tight makes you feel extra tingly. If you're able to balance without resting your hands on your man's legs, free them up to explore his balls and perineum. The added sensation will drive him crazy and hasten his climax.

WHAT'S IN IT FOR HIM

It could be difficult for you to maintain this position for long, but it won't matter, because the unique angle of penetration combined with her vagina's warm and tight caress will have you ready to explode before long. When an upper-body strength workout becomes this delicious, you may end up exchanging your gym membership for extra private "training" sessions with her!

Choose Your Own Erotic Adventure

Need to build up to LAP OF LUXURY? Attending Hatha or power yoga lessons together will limber you both up and introduce you to backbends and the kind of breathing techniques necessary to hold these positions. In the meantime, you can enjoy a variation of this position where the man is seated and the woman lowers herself into his lap in the same manner. Better yet, try both and compare notes to see how the sensations differ and decide which makes it into your sex recipe box.

No. 32
PRIME RIB

Make mine medium rare.

HOW TO

This is similar to Position #8 (SLICE OF HEAVEN, page 29), except that the man gets to be in control! She kneels on the bed, with her torso lowered and her arms extended in front of you. He is also kneeling, but upright. He positions himself behind her, between her legs, and enters her from behind, grabbing her waist to pull her into him with each lusty thrust!

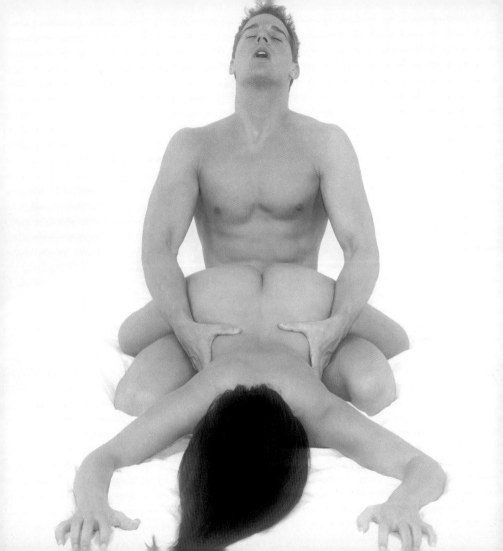

WHAT'S IN IT FOR HER

In this position, he's perfectly angled to hit your oh-so-sensitive G-spot! Placing cushions underneath your pelvis will enhance your excitement as each thrust will create feel-good friction on your clitoris.

WHAT'S IN IT FOR HIM

That view! Her ass and back are on a platter for you to admire, and you're open to devour her as you please . . . You can grab and fondle her backside, or massage and lightly scratch her back. If you're both feeling especially frisky, you can gently tug on her hair or push her arms down so that she is pinned down. In this easy-to-maneuver position, a little imagination goes a long way toward making a tame lovemaking session unforgettable!

Fantasy Island

There's not a lot of opportunity for intimacy in this position, because you can't see each other's faces, so why not explore playing out your fantasies? Imagine yourself with another hottie, and encourage your man to do the same!

This can end up being an extremely erotic experiment, and one that can actually deepen your relationship. By sharing each other's innermost sexual desires, you show that you trust your partner and it provides an opportunity for each of you to learn more about what gets you hot!

No. 33
VALUABLE
ASSETS

Getting to the bottom of it.

HOW TO

With this variation on traditional woman-on-top sex, she gets a fun way to begin exploring the many pleasures that can be found when she and her partner turn their attention to her ass. When they're both primed for action, she climbs on top of him, and places his hands firmly on her butt cheeks. Although he probably won't need the encouragement, she can entice him to focus on her hind region with a verbal torrent of sexy commands.

Be sure to be equally vocal about what feels good!

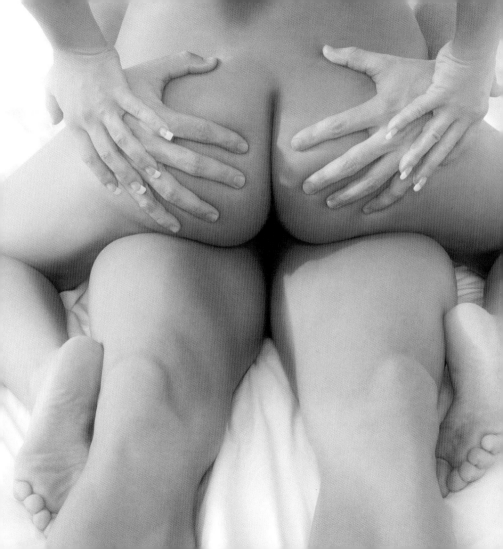

�֍ WHAT'S IN IT FOR HER

No matter what kind of hang-ups you might have with your ass, when your partner plays with it you'll soon forget any insecurities you have and get lost in how good it feels! In fact, inviting your man to explore your body in this way goes a long way toward becoming more comfortable in your own skin.

✖ WHAT'S IN IT FOR HIM

Many women derive intense pleasure from having their ass grabbed, massaged, and lightly pinched, scratched, or slapped! (For the latter, just make sure you talk about whether you're both OK with rougher play . . .) This type of ass-attention will likely fulfill some wild fantasies for both of you!

No. 34
RANDY ROULETTE

This could be your lucky number!

HOW TO

Here's a daring position that requires a bit of coordination on the part of both lovers. Unlike an actual roulette wheel, the spinning motion here needs to be slow and controlled. This is not for the sexually inexperienced, but with some practice, it's easy to master—and once you do, you'll feel like you hit the jackpot!

She lies on the bed with arms by her side and legs slightly parted. For best results, place a pillow under her to tilt her pelvis up for easier penetration. He is in missionary position, but facing the opposite direction, so his head is at

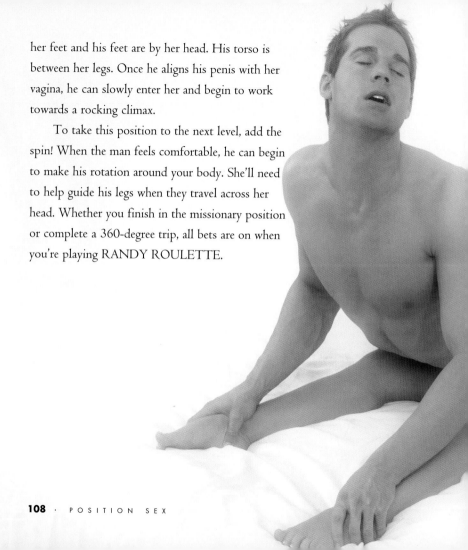

her feet and his feet are by her head. His torso is between her legs. Once he aligns his penis with her vagina, he can slowly enter her and begin to work towards a rocking climax.

To take this position to the next level, add the spin! When the man feels comfortable, he can begin to make his rotation around your body. She'll need to help guide his legs when they travel across her head. Whether you finish in the missionary position or complete a 360-degree trip, all bets are on when you're playing RANDY ROULETTE.

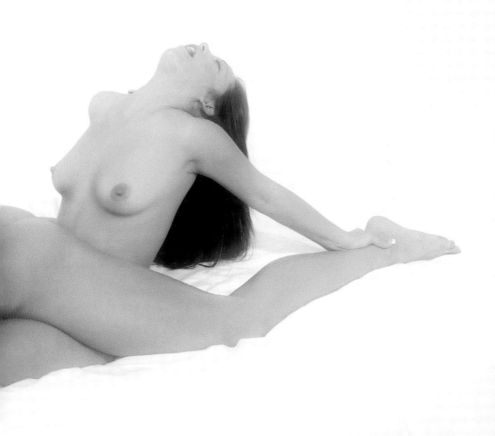

✖ WHAT'S IN IT FOR HER

Although this is not as intimate as other positions, you can still maintain contact with your man by either sitting up and leaning back on his legs, or by lying down and grasping his buttocks. The upside is that you get a unique view of your man's bod, and aside from needing to coordinate during penetration and during the spin cycle, you don't need to exert a lot of energy.

✖ WHAT'S IN IT FOR HIM

This is a prime opportunity for you to show off your agility! Shallow thrusting means that the focus of penetration is on the sensitive head of your penis— always a good thing for you! And an added blissful benefit for both is that your balls will rub against her vagina, something that feels great and doesn't always occur in tamer entanglements.

No. 35
HELLO DOLLY!

She's armed for action.

HOW TO

She positions herself on all fours either on the bed or on the floor. He stands behind, and slowly grabs onto her legs and lifts them up so that they are level with his hips. At this point, she'll be doing a modified handstand! He'll then part her legs so he can enter her from behind in this novel position. He should have a firm grasp on her upper thighs; for added feelings of support (and for leverage when pumping), wrap the lower part of her legs around his ass.

✂ WHAT'S IN IT FOR HER

Here's one advantage to having toned arms that the trainer neglected to share with you! This position requires serious arm strength. If you're up for the challenge, you won't be disappointed! Penetration is deep in this position and the angle is such that you should get a serious G-spot massage! If your man is not extremely well-endowed, this position will make him feel bigger. You'll also get the sensation of a rush of blood to the head, which some women love! However, if at any point you feel dizzy, you should stop—fainting during sex is sure to kill the mood.

✖ WHAT'S IN IT FOR HIM

You are in absolute control of the rhythm, and pretty much anything goes! You can try circular or up-and-down motions, or you can squeeze your legs together then open them up . . . . She can heighten the sensations by squeezing her PC muscles slowly and gently.

Since men are visual creatures, you'll definitely enjoy the view from above! Your lover can act out as much as possible by gyrating against you while also giving you a running commentary about her bobbing breasts and throbbing clitoris. In this position, they're out of your line of vision and impossible to fondle, but her sultry descriptions will go a long way toward fueling your hungry imagination.

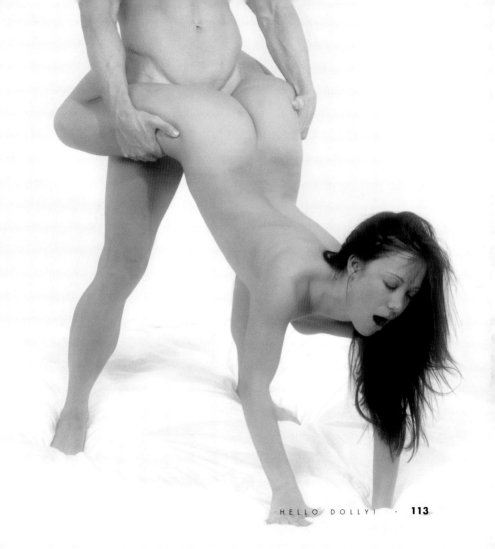

No. 36
SPOONFUL OF SUGAR

A sweet retreat.

HOW TO

For those quieter times when you want to savor your partner in a more deliberate and loving manner, this position is a must. She lies on her side in front of her man, and parts her legs slightly so he can push his erect penis into her from behind. Slowly rock to orgasm while focusing on the warm feeling of his hands exploring every inch of her body.

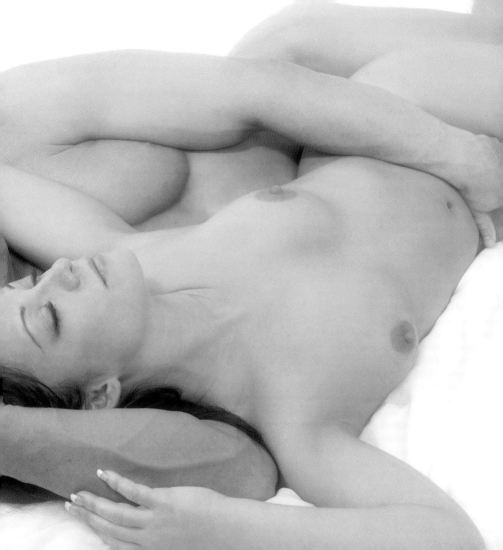

✂ WHAT'S IN IT FOR HER

This highly intimate position allows him to express his feelings for you through slow and sensuous caressing. A woman's neck is a highly erogenous area of her body, and when he's nuzzled up next to you while spooning, he's perfectly situated to tease, lick, and kiss this sensitive and oft-ignored area.

✼ WHAT'S IN IT FOR HIM

All of this touching sends a rush of feel-good chemicals to the pleasure center of your brain. By spending time exploring her body, you become intimately acquainted with what she likes and what you like even more! Tell her not to be shy when it comes to telling you which buttons to push and where to let your hands linger.

Choose Your Own Erotic Adventure

It can also be hot to avoid penetration altogether, in lieu of touching each other until you can't take it any more! This spooning position is suited to this kind of amped-up foreplay, in that you are able to touch, kiss, and caress each other until the heat rises to the point of no return. There's also a lot of skin-on-skin contact. Set up parameters of what's off-limits, and see how long you can each hold out. You'll find that as you attempt to refrain from intercourse, you want it more! If you submit to the urge, you're in for an off-the-Richter-scale orgasm!

No. 37
ROCKING HORSE

Rockabye ... oh, boy!

HOW TO

When you're in the mood for a G-spot special, the ROCKING HORSE delivers. Start out with him kneeling on the bed with his legs bent underneath him. (If his knees bother him, he can extend his slightly bent legs out in front of him, instead.) Facing him, she sits down on his lap with her feet on the bed and guides his hard penis into her vagina. He grasps her back to support her. She leans her hands back on the bed for extra support, and slowly brings her legs up to rest on his shoulders. She either remains leaning back, or grabs hold of his forearms. Sync your rhythm so that you're moving back and forth together.

✂ WHAT'S IN IT FOR HER

He's not likely to come too quickly in this position, so he's free to focus on your pleasure! If you feel supported enough with one arm behind you, he can free up a hand to massage your clitoris, adding to your excitement. Motion in this position is somewhat limited, so to maintain penetration, your man needs to gently roll his hips and sway forward and back.

❄ WHAT'S IN IT FOR HIM

You'll direct the movement and she'll rely on your strength to keep you both balanced and in sync. You'll hold out for a long time, which makes you feel like a stud! If she wants to make this a more amped-up sex session, she can lean back with her hands on the bed. This will allow you to thrust deeper.

Choose Your Own Erotic Adventure—for Her

Feeling really crazy? Make an adjustment to the position: Instead of leaning your hands back, hook your arms around your man's neck so that you're in a more compact configuration, and take this position to a rocking chair! Of course, if you move too much, you risk falling and hurting yourself—let the chair do the rocking for you!

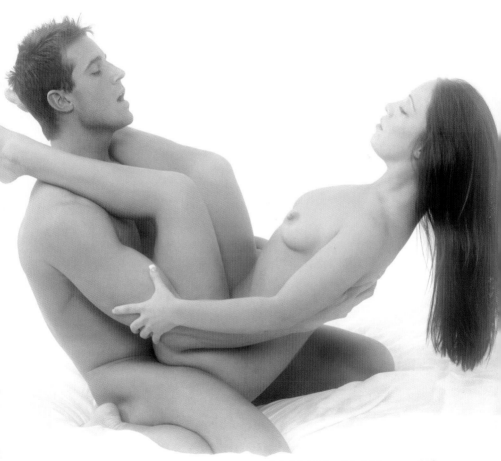

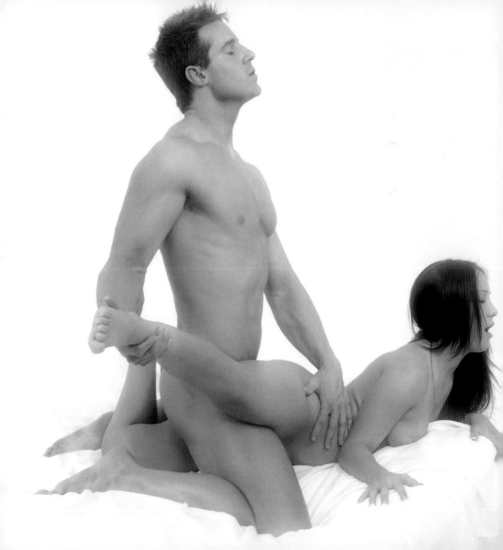

No. 38
CARNAL CROSSBOW

His weapon of choice.

HOW TO

She lies on her stomach on the bed while he positions himself between her legs—they're parted like scissors. He's kneeling and straddling one of her legs. As he enters her from behind, he lifts her other leg so that it's fully extended. He supports her leg at the ankle while also placing a hand on her hip to direct his love arrow!

WHAT'S IN IT FOR HER

If you're prone to get off on feeling submissive, this is a good position to try! He will be in total control, driving the motion, thrusting, and tempo. There's a slight angle to penetration and thrusting will be somewhat shallow, so you're in for a treat! Areas of your vagina that aren't normally stimulated will get some attention in the CARNAL CROSSBOW. For additional lusty leverage, push off the side of the bed and grind into your man's pelvis.

WHAT'S IN IT FOR HIM

Your virility is on display as you go in for the kill. You can adjust her leg height according to what feels best, and pull her into you with some force to fulfill your animal urges. This position lends itself to some serious role playing—a knight/damsel medieval romp, a rockstar/groupie fantasy, a Tarzan/Jane scenario . . . . Let your imagination take you to unprecedented heights. You'll hold out for a long time in this position, so play with it!

Love You Long Time

Originating in 3000 B.C.E., Tantric sex techniques allow intercourse to last for hours. Start with thrusting in patterns: nine fast, deep ones, then one slow, shallow one; then eight deep, then two shallow; then seven deep and so on. Those old guys really knew their stuff, their shallow thrusts were honing in on her G-spot five thousand years before any scientist was able to locate it.

No. 39
FOLD & FONDLE

Over stimulated ...

HOW TO

Although FOLD & FONDLE provides a mellow alternative to some of the more energetic positions presented here, it's no less satisfying and makes for a great addition to your lovemaking lineup. Begin with the man sitting upright on the bed with his legs outstretched in front of him. She sits in his lap, onto his erect penis, and then slowly leans forward. He folds forward with her, as if the two of them are riding together in a toboggan. The motion is very gentle; virtually devoid of thrusting. Make waves by focusing on small, but stimulating circular gyrations and pulsing PC contractions. It may seem simple, but don't underestimate the power of subtle application of pressure! Sync up your breathing for a relaxing and spiritual experience.

✻ WHAT'S IN IT FOR HER

Craving intimacy? You get it here. With your man cuddled in close, you get extra skin-time, causing an all-over buzz. He can also reach around and lavish your breasts with much-deserved attention. You call the shots, so tease him by squeezing and contracting your pelvic floor—the sensation will drive him wild! Wait to see his reaction!

✖ WHAT'S IN IT FOR HIM

When she leans forward, your penis gets a squeeze, which warms you up all over. Add to that the pleasure of her gripping your throbbing member and it'll be almost too much for you to handle! She'll send you to the moon by fondling your testicles (especially if she remembers to massage and apply pressure to your oh-so-sensitive perineum). The lack of movement in this position means you're free to caress her breasts and lavish her back with kisses.

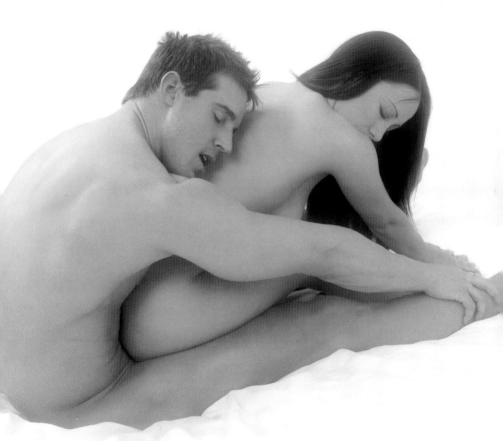

No. 40
TIDAL WAVE

Surf's up!

HOW TO

The woman lies on the bed, propping herself up on her elbows with her legs open wide. (For easier penetration, she might want to slide a pillow beneath her.) He faces away from her and positions himself on all fours, bringing his legs on either side of her torso. Once he's comfortable, he can guide his penis into her vagina. Getting the angle right might take a little practice, so be sure to help each other out by communicating throughout. This entanglement is pretty advanced, so make sure you two relish in your sexual adventurousness!

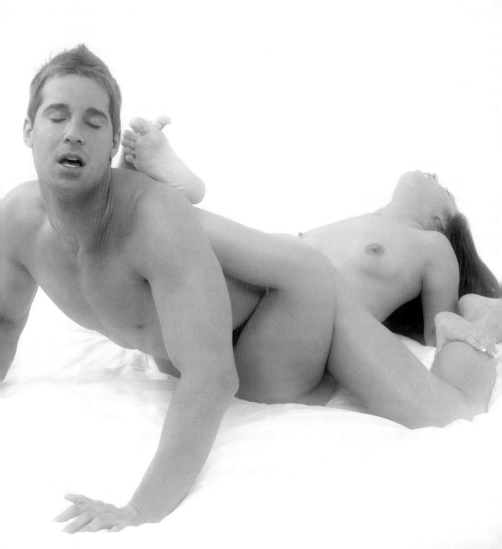

✂ WHAT'S IN IT FOR HER

Although intimacy is out of the question in this position, you'll receive ample stimulation in your midsection as your clitoris and lips are in full contact with your man's pelvis and the area around his penis. The sensations concentrated around your vagina will be intense! When you use your feet and arms as leverage to pull your man in deeper, you'll be riding the big kahuna in no time!

✖ WHAT'S IN IT FOR HIM

Embrace the rip curl for the best results (read: circular movements will get you far!). The inability to see each other makes this position exciting, as does the novelty of receiving unexpected caresses.

Sex, Al Fresco

Next time you're at the beach, why not consider getting it on? Communing with nature in the truest sense, there's something inherently delicious about *al fresco* sex. Perhaps it's the feeling of having fresh air kiss your naked body or the freedom of losing yourself in elements and your lover at the same time. Either way, having sex in the wild is a great way to elevate your pleasure to another level.

No. 41
SIDE SADDLE

Hot to trot!

HOW TO

He lies on his back, with both legs slightly bent and pointing upward. She straddles his body sideways, mounting his erect penis in doing so. She uses his knees to keep herself stable. She turns her back slightly so that it is angled toward his face, and she takes him out for one wild ride!

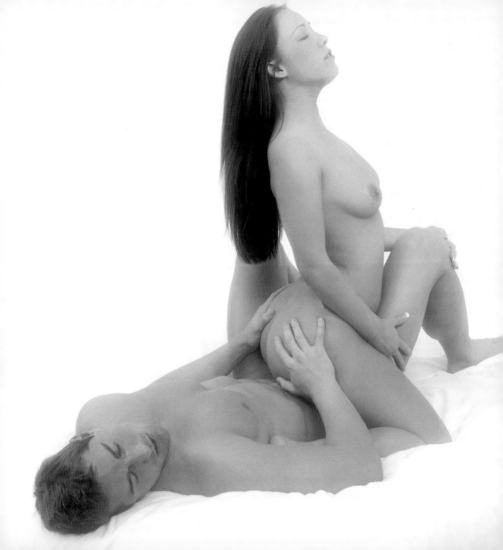

✖ WHAT'S IN IT FOR HER

You take hold of the reins in this lusty woman-on-top configuration! You adjust the tempo, depth of thrusting, and motion, so feel free to get creative! Try teasing him by pulling yourself up high, so that his penis is almost all the way out of your vagina, hovering with the head at the entrance, circling around, and then plunging deep. Or, gyrate for a minute then switch to quick up-and-down movements, then go deep. Squeeze your PC muscles intermittently, and rub your breasts into his legs. Go with whatever feels good to you—you can get a thrill out of keeping him guessing. Ride him cowgirl!

✖ WHAT'S IN IT FOR HIM

You get to lie back and enjoy the ride! If you're feeling frisky, you can raise your pelvis to add a little bucking action to the romp, but otherwise, you can just relish in the view of her bobbing ass. She's directing this horse, and you're going wherever she points you. The two of you can go far in this SIDE SADDLE.

No. 42
SIZZLING SCISSORS

A cut above.

HOW TO

She lies with her back so that her ass is in line with the edge of the bed. She holds her legs up straight in the air. He kneels at the foot of the bed, and can place a pillow underneath his knees for a comfier ride, as well as adjust the height so that he can easily penetrate her. After entering her wet vagina, he grabs her legs, crosses them, and holds them in front of his face. He continues to crisscross her legs throughout the SIZZLING SCISSORS sex session!

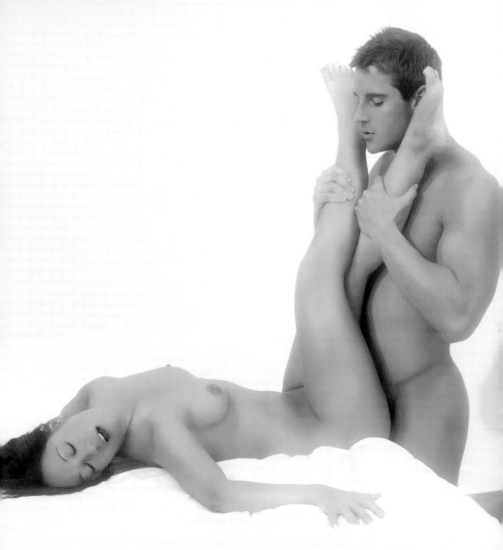

✄ WHAT'S IN IT FOR HER

The yummy sensations of your vagina squeezed tight, alternated with the deep thrusting when you're spread wide open, sends a chill up your supine spine. Allow your hands to travel to your breasts or your clitoris for additional tactile pleasures. (See sidebar.)

✖ WHAT'S IN IT FOR HIM

If you're a leg-man, this is a terrific position for you to take in her gorgeous gams. If you're a breast man, you have a perfect view of them and can tease her and up the temperature by telling her exactly what you'd like to do with them (e.g., fondle, bite, lick, pinch)! If you're lucky, she'll provide extra sensory stimulus by playing with herself. You'll enjoy the athletic crisscross maneuvering required to pump your penis until it's perfectly primed for climax.

How She Can Tit-illate Him

With free hands, this position is perfectly suited to you giving your man a show by fondling your breasts! Gently touch your breasts and note how they feel—smooth, heavy, light, full, slim . . . . Trace the shape and continue to lightly fondle them. Note the sensations verbally or with a low moan to get a rise out of your guy.

No. 43
MAKE A WISH

History-making oral.

HOW TO

During a heated session in the sack, she pretends she is a genie, and assumes her man has wished for a mind-blowing climax! She starts by spoiling him with an all-over body massage with special oil to relax him and release tension in his tight muscles. He lies on his stomach, and she lavishes his back, ass, and legs with attention. She can vary the pressure, and ask him what he likes best! He then flips over and she begins by massaging his chest in a sensuous and drawn-out fashion to build up to the main event! Eventually she inches down to his pelvic region, where she'll focus her erotic energies on making his dream(s) come true!

✄ WHAT'S IN IT FOR HER
You get to deliver a blissful treat!

✄ WHAT'S IN IT FOR HIM
You receive a delicious memory that will linger in your mind—and on your body!

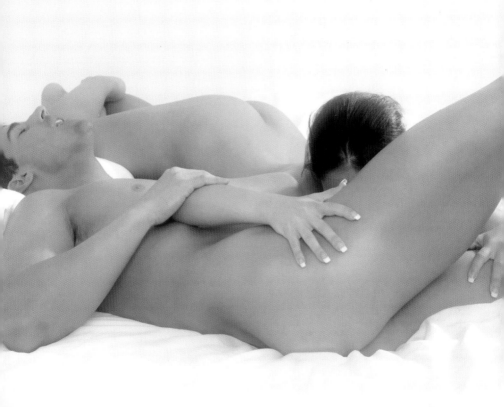

No. 44
QUEEN
FOR A DAY

The royal treatment.

HOW TO

When he lavishes her with this kind of attention, she'll wonder who died and made her queen! She sets the tone with a few royal commands (namely, "Don't dive straight for my clitoris!") but then lets him create the erotic scene. He'll evoke a sensual mood with candles, pillows, and aphrodisiacs or oils. He'll spend time kissing her lips, breasts, and belly. He'll stroke her lightly with his fingertips and tell her how beautiful she is. Only after she's feeling relaxed and primed for it, he'll move down between her legs and gently blow, stroke, and nibble his way to her forbidden fruit.

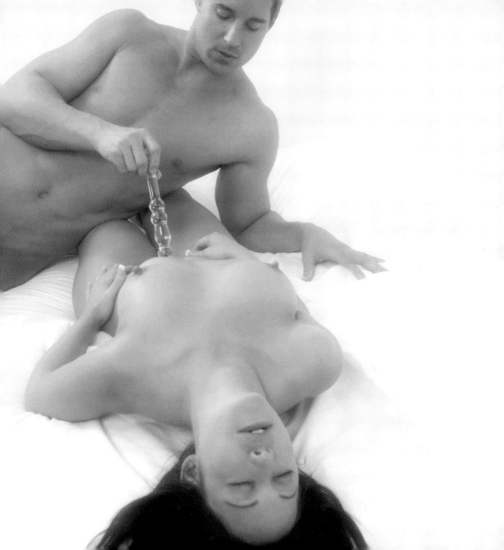

Your every wish is his command.

You become a valued member of the court's "inner circle."

Oral Techniques (for Her Pleasure)

Again, every woman has different likes and dislikes when it comes to her man performing oral sex. But with some dedication, you will quickly come to realize the special areas and techniques that drive her wild. Here are some guidelines to get you started:

- The clitoris has more nerve endings than the entire head of the penis—be gentle!
- Tell her how good she looks, smells, and tastes.
- Know where the clitoris is, but don't dive straight for it; first try kissing and licking around the upper thighs and vulva.
- Ask her what she likes. She'll at least say "harder," "slower," or "more circles."
- Think variety—if you repeat the same motion, she may become insensitive to it, so be sure to vary your stimulation.
- As she becomes more aroused, insert a finger or two into her vagina and experiment with motions and applying pressure.
- Unlike men, many women enjoy strong stimulation while having an orgasm. Keep it going until she asks you to stop.
- Continue to fondle and hold her as she orgasms and bask in her afterglow.

No. 45
BEDTIME STORIES

A naughty nightcap.

HOW TO

Have your fantasies ready to share, because it's confession time! While crouching on the bed, he enters her from behind, a la Position #5 (RUMP ROMP, page 20) and covers her with his hot bod. As his captive audience, he's free to titillate her with his innermost desires.

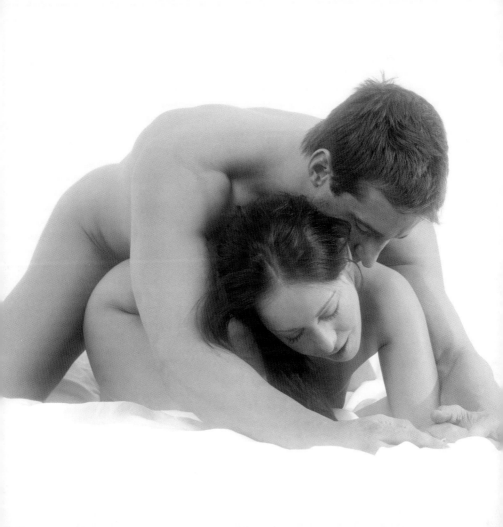

❊ WHAT'S IN IT FOR HER

Hot sex with the added jolt that comes with sharing something as intimate as a fantasy.

❊ WHAT'S IN IT FOR HIM

You can begin to broach the subject of kinkier sex in a way that will make you more willing to experiment.

Fantasy Rank

According to a poll of six thousand men and women conducted by the editors of *Cosmopolitan* and *Men's Health* in early 2006, the top fantasies for both sexes are as follows:

WOMEN

1. She's trapped in a burning building, he's a fireman.
2. She's in trouble, he's a police officer.
3. She's a student, he's a professor.

MEN

1. He's a patient, she's a nurse.
2. He's a student, she's a professor.
3. He's a professor, she's a student.

No. 46
X-GAMES

Climbing the walls ...

HOW TO

A little dexterity goes a long way toward adding spice to your sex life—this position is a testament to that. He lies down with only his head, shoulders, and upper back on the bed; his legs are upright and leaning against the wall. She positions herself so that her back is to him, and using the wall for support, squats onto his erect penis. The penetration needs to be controlled, but then he can grasp her ass and get down to the thrusting action.

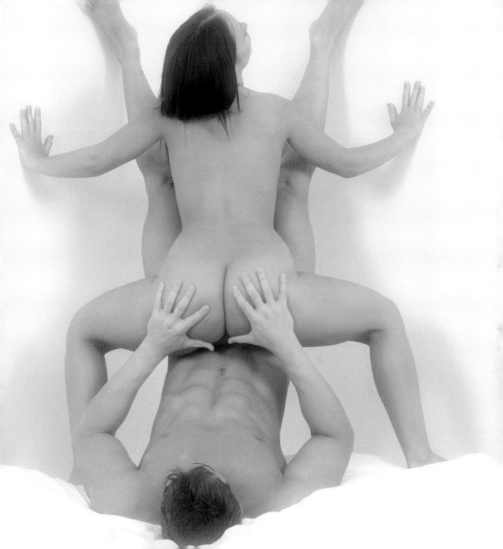

WHAT'S IN IT FOR HER

Show off your hot bod, as he feels you up in any way that he pleases! In this position, his penis rubs against the front of your vaginal wall, where the elusive G-spot lives, meaning you're in for super-stimulation. Because you're standing, you're in the driver's seat, and thrusting is easy. Grind your bottom half into your man, then reach for his balls. He won't know what hit him!

WHAT'S IN IT FOR HIM

You've got to work a little harder than you would if you were in a prone position, but the view and the tingly sensations from the inversion make it all worthwhile. You'll get an abdominals workout in the process.

Stand and Deliver

One problem with stand-up sex is that there's often a difference between your heights. That doesn't make sex of the vertical variety impossible—it just means you may need to make modifications.

- Take the stairs. If you're shorter, have him stand on flat ground while you stand on the first step.
- Stand face-to-face and have the man bend his knees slightly so he can penetrate her.
- She wraps her arms and legs around him while he lifts her up. If he gets tired, he can lean her against a wall to help carry the weight.
- Break out a pair of stilettos. There's no better excuse to sport a sexy pair of high heels in the bedroom.

No. 47
OVER
THE EDGE

The floor model.

HOW TO

She lies facedown, leaning over the edge of the bed; one leg rests on the floor, the other leg is outstretched. He gets into the same position, on top of her, and enters her from behind for a steamy half-on, half-off the bed romp.

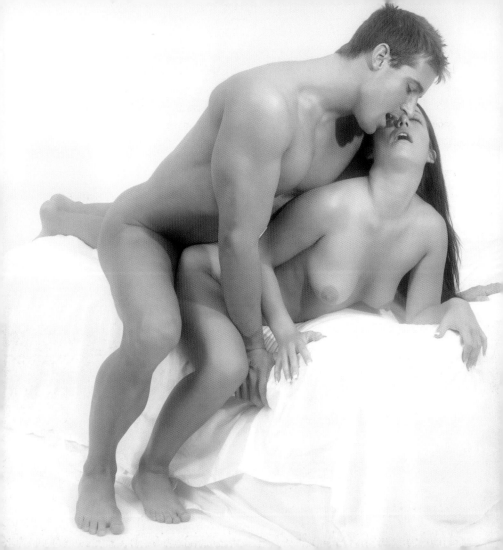

✂ WHAT'S IN IT FOR HER

Ideal for vigorous sex and deep penetration, with the added benefit of having leverage of a foot on the floor to thrust even more energetically! His penis will hit your all-important G-spot, and the animalistic nature of this sexual experience will rev both of your engines for kinkier fare. Even the most mild-mannered guy usually lets loose when he's sent OVER THE EDGE.

✠ WHAT'S IN IT FOR HIM

The ultimate position of control, you'll like this because you feel a sense of domination. You'll enjoy the feeling of your balls slapping against her. You also get to see all of the action, which includes a sweet view of her swinging breasts.

Intro to Anal Play

Guys, curious about anal play, but not sure where to start? Well, first and foremost, make sure you have an open dialogue with your partner about your interest and never (read: *never*) try to spring a surprise entry on her. It may take some time for her to warm up to the idea.

Despite the taboo around them, you may find the use of anal toys to be extremely stimulating and with patience, time, and a relaxed environment they can bring great pleasure to your sex life. Anal toys, such as butt plugs and anal beads, are designed to be inserted in to the anal cavity and stimulate the nerves surrounding the anus.

No. 48
SPLITTING WOOD

A treehugger's pose.

HOW TO

She lies on her back on the bed with one leg raised high in the air. He straddles her leg, enters her, and rests her raised leg on his chest. (A pillow under her ass will give him a better angle to guide his penis into her vagina, and help him achieve deeper penetration.) In this position, he can use her leg as an exciting way to leverage the many hot and heavy thrusting possibilities.

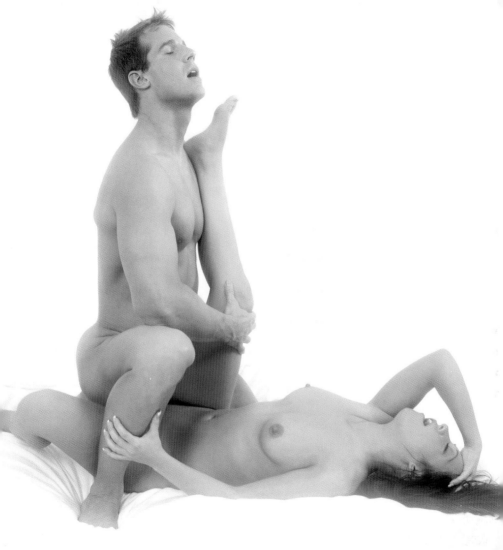

✴ WHAT'S IN IT FOR HER

Got sexy legs? Here's where you can show them off! Feeling extra limber from your three-times a week yoga practice? Here's the big payoff. This position allows you to really flaunt your flexibility, athleticism, and sexiness. Pamper your feet before engaging in SPLITTING WOOD, your man will have an up-close view of your tootsies. A bonus if he's got a thing for feet.

✴ WHAT'S IN IT FOR HIM

You're in control in this lusty leg-raiser! You'll be thrilled at the deep penetration that is possible, as well as turned on by the view of your erect penis disappearing into her wet vagina and then emerging again. You can grab her ass to pull her into you as your bodies meet during thrusting. This is one position where he can let his animalistic side roam free.

Toe Turn-On

Why not spoil each other with a sexy foot massage? According to the principles of reflexology, stimulating points on the feet can result in beneficial effects on some other parts of the body and will improve your general health. A foot massage can bring rejuvenation to your body. Start with a bath of lightly scented salts, then pat each other's feet dry with a warm, fluffy towel. Take time to rub your lover's feet with oils, kneading each toe gently. When you're through, feelings of relaxation should wash over you both.

No. 49
UP & AWAY

A swingers's delight.

HOW TO

In this position, he remains standing. She wraps her arms around his neck, and with help from him, she wraps her legs around his waist, in the process of lining her vagina up with his penis so that he can enter her. This obviously requires strength and coordination on the part of lovers, so maneuvering into this position is slow and controlled. Once she's comfortably penetrated, let the swinging begin!

WHAT'S IN IT FOR HER

Having your man carry you in his arms can be a powerful turn-on for a woman! Sex in this position can also lend itself to very romantic feelings. You'll feel an intimate bond with your lover as you cling to him with each swinging thrust and make eye contact.

WHAT'S IN IT FOR HIM

You'll relish the animalistic nature of UP & AWAY! It also affords you the deep penetration that you've come to love. This is one position where you can show off your strength and prowess. It's got the duality of being intimate and being primal; the perfect combination to satisfy both partners.

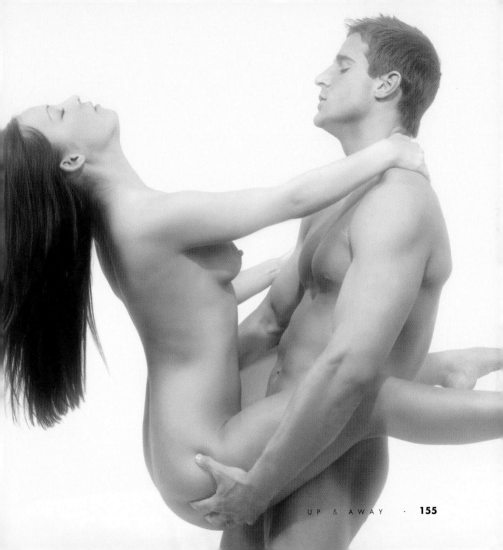

No. 50
CROSSLEG
CANOODLE

Ready to rock your world.

HOW TO

This position begins as a tangle of limbs and ends in rhythmic bliss. She starts out by straddling her man who's on his back. Her legs should be bent and her feet flat on the bed. She slides on to his erect penis. Once they're joined, he should slowly sit upright and bend his knees so that they are pointed slightly outward at a 45-degree angle. She matches his leg position, and weaves her arms underneath his knees so that her hands are resting on his thighs. He should do the same, but his arms come under her knees and rest on her back for support. Hold the position for a minute and then get in sync and rock away!

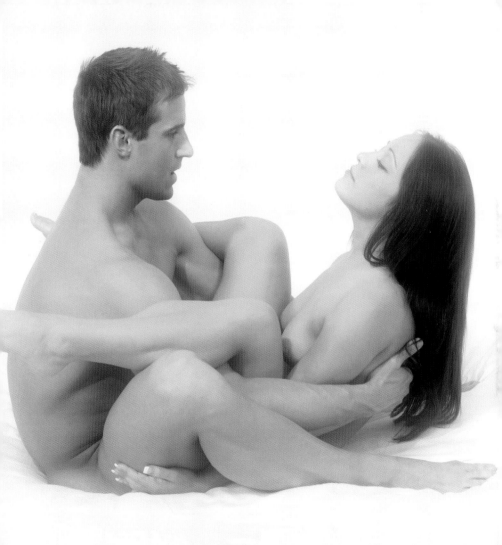

WHAT'S IN IT FOR HER

Because the CROSSLEG CANOODLE is better suited to shallow penetration, your man can wake up the nerve endings in the first third of your vagina while stimulating the ultra-sensitive head of his penis—a treat for you both!

WHAT'S IN IT FOR HIM

Lots of skin contact gets you feeling tingly all-over. You'll savor the wonderful close-up view of her body rubbing next to yours! Since deep thrusting might cause you to lose penetration, she should treat you to some well-timed squeezes of her PC muscles for added penile pleasure! Pulling her closer to kiss and nuzzle her neck will elevate the experience to unforgettable.

Sex Matters!

More and more studies tout the increased emotional and physical benefits from frequent safe sex. With this many good things to come out of it, it's only logical that you continue to explore this sacred union with your lover—if for nothing else, then for your health!

- Lowers mortality rates
- Reduces the risk of prostate cancer
- Reduces the risk of heart disease
- Offers pain-relief
- Improves posture
- Increases self-esteem
- Makes people feel younger
- Makes people feel more calm
- Gives people a positive attitude on life
- Reduces incidents of depression
- Improves sense of smell
- Firms tummy and buttocks
- Improves fitness level
- Keeps lovers connected emotionally

A B O U T   T H E   A U T H O R

LOLA RAWLINS has edited several sex books related to harnessing sexual energy and taking it for a ride. She has been researching creative positions for years and counts on trying a new one tonight and hope you do, too. Lola lives in Pawtucket, Rhode Island.